GEOMETRICAL
AND
VISUAL OPTICS

NOTICE

GEOMETRICAL
AND
VISUAL OPTICS

A Clinical Introduction

Steven H. Schwartz, OD, PhD

Vice President and Dean for Academic Affairs
State University of New York
State College of Optometry
New York, New York

McGraw-Hill
Medical Publishing Division

New York Chicago San Francisco Lisbon London Madrid
Mexico City Milan New Delhi San Juan Seoul
Singapore Sydney Toronto

McGraw-Hill

A Division of The McGraw·Hill Companies

GEOMETRICAL AND VISUAL OPTICS: A Clinical Introduction

1234567890 DOC/DOC 098765432

ISBN 0-07-137415-9

This book was set in Garamond by Hightstown Desktop Publishing.
The editors were Darlene Barela Cooke and Lester A. Sheinis.
The production manager was Phil Galea.
The illustration manager was Charissa Baker.
The cover designer was Aimée Nordin.
The indexer was Alexandra Nickerson.
R. R. Donnelley & Sons Company was printer and binder.

This book is printed on acid-free paper.

Library of Congress Cataloging-in-Publication Data

Schwartz, Steven H.
    Geometrical and visual optics / Steven H. Schwatrz.
      p. ; cm.
    Includes bibliographical references and index.
    ISBN 0-07-137415-9
    1. Physiological optics. 2. Geometrical optics. I. Title.
    [DNLM: 1. Optics—Problems and Exercises. 2. Lenses—Problems and Exercises. 3. Refraction, Ocular—Problems and Exercises. 4. Vision—Problems and Exercises. WW 18.2 S399g 2002]
    QP475 .S379 2002
    617.7'5'076—dc21
                                        2001044815

Contents

Preface xi

1. Basic Terms and Concepts 1
  • Objects, Light Rays, and Pencils 2
  • Vergence 4
  • Refraction 5
  • Snell's Law 6
  • Self-Assessment Problems 12

2. Refraction at Spherical Surfaces 13
  • Converging and Diverging Surfaces 13
  • More on Focal Points 16
  • Refracting Power and Focal Lengths 18
  • Another Way to Calculate Power 19
  • Real Images 21
  • Virtual Images 22
  • Self-Assessment Problems 24

3. The Vergence Relationship 27
  • Basic Concepts 27
  • More on Vergence 28
  • Sign Conventions 31
  • Sample Problems 32
    Converging Surface 32
    Location of Focal Points 35
    Diverging Surface 35
    Locating the Object When Given the Image Location 37

Surface with No Power 38
• Self-Assessment Problems 41

4. Thin Lenses **43**
• Focal Points 43
• Ray Tracing 47
• Paraxial Relationship 47
• Newton's Relation 50
• Self-Assessment Problems 52

5. Optical Systems with Multiple Surfaces **53**
• Multiple Thin Lens Systems 53
• Virtual Objects 57
• Thick Lenses 59
• Self-Assessment Problems 62

6. Equivalent Lenses **63**
• Definitions and Formulae 63
Equivalent Power 65
Front Vertex and Back Vertex Power 66
Principal Planes 67
• Sample Problem 67
• Locating an Image Using an Equivalent Lens 72
• Nodal Points 73
• Self-Assessment Problems 75

7. Schematic Eyes and Ametropia **77**
• Gullstrand and Reduced Eye Models 77
• Emmetropia 79
• Myopia 80
• Hyperopia 82
• Far-Point in Emmetropia 85
• Far-Point Vergence Relationship 85
• Lens Effectivity 87
• Correction of Ametropia with Laser and Surgical Procedures 90
• Self-Assessment Problems 94

8. Accommodation **95**
• Accommodation in the Emmetropic Eye 96
• Accommodation in Uncorrected Ametropia 98
• Near Point of Accommodation 101
• Accommodation in Corrected Ametropia .103
• Correction of Presbyopia 108
• Self-Assessment Problems 111

9. Cylindrical Lenses and the Correction of Astigmatism 113
- Lens Crosses 114
- Lens Formulae/Prescriptions 116
- Image Formation: Point Sources 119
- Image Formation: Extended Sources .121
- Astigmatism: Definitions and Classifications 123
- Jackson Crossed-Cylinder Test 126
- Spherical Equivalency 127
- What Does the Astigmat See? 129
- Self-Assessment Problems 131

10. Prisms 133
- Angle of Deviation 133
- Prism Power 135
- Prismatic Effects of Lenses 137
- Prentice's Rule 137
- Clinical Applications 140
- Self-Assessment Problems 144

11. Depth of Field 145
- Blur Circles and Visual Acuity 145
- Depth of Field and Depth of Focus 150
- Hyperfocal Distance 154
- Self-Assessment Problems 157

12. Magnifying Devices 159
- Magnification by Plus Lenses 159
  - Lateral Magnification 159
  - Effective Magnification 160
  - Angular Magnification of a Plus Lens 162
  - The Problem with Magnification 163
- Prescribing Near-Plus Magnifiers 163
  - Magnifying Lens and Bifocal Add in Combination 166
  - Fixed-Focus Stand Magnifiers 167
  - Closed-Circuit Television 170
  - More on Near Magnification Devices 170
- Telescopes 170
  - Galilean Telescopes 171
  - Keplerian Telescopes 171
  - An Alternative Method of Determining a Telescope's
    Angular Magnification 173
  - Lens Caps 174
- Self-Assessment Problems 177

13. Retinal Image Size **179**
   • Linear Size of the Retinal Image in Uncorrected Ametropia 179
   • Spectacle Magnification 181
   • Angular Magnification in Corrected Ametropia 183
   • Physical Image Size in Corrected Ametropia 184
   • Summary 187
   • Self-Assessment Problems 189

14. Reflection **191**
   • Ray Tracing: Concave, Convex, and Plane Mirrors 191
      Concave Mirrors 191
      Convex Mirrors 193
      Plane Mirrors. 195
   • Power of Mirrors 196
   • The Vergence (Paraxial) Relationship 198
   • Reflections and Antireflective Coatings 203
   • Purkinje Images 206
      Location of Purkinje Image I 207
      Location of Purkinje Image III 209
   • Corneal Topography 213
   • Keratometry and Contact Lenses 214
   • Javal's Rule 219
   • Self-Assessment Problems 223

15. Aberrations **225**
   • The Paraxial Assumption 225
   • Seidel Aberrations 226
      Spherical Aberration 227
      Coma 229
      Radial Astigmatism 234
      Curvature of Field 235
      Distortion. 236
   • Spherical Aberration of the Human Eye 237
   • Wavefront Sensing and Adaptive Optics 237
      Measurement of the Eye's Monochromatic Aberrations 238
      Supernormal Vision. 240
      Imaging the Fundus. 242
   • Chromatic Aberrations 243
      Dispersive Power and Constrigence 244
      Achromatic Lenses 245
   • Chromatic Aberrations of the Human Eye .247
   • The Red-Green Refraction Technique 249
   • Lateral (Transverse) Chromatic Aberration 249
   • Self-Assessment Problems 252

Answers to Self-Assessment Problems 253
  • Chapter 1   Basic Terms and Concepts 253
  • Chapter 2   Refraction at Spherical Surfaces 254
  • Chapter 3   The Vergence Relationship 256
  • Chapter 4   Thin Lenses 260
  • Chapter 5   Optical Systems with Multiple Surfaces 262
  • Chapter 6   Equivalent Lenses 268
  • Chapter 7   Schematic Eyes and Ametropia 275
  • Chapter 8   Accommodation 278
  • Chapter 9   Cylindrical Lenses and the Correction of Astigmatism . .282
  • Chapter 10   Prisms 287
  • Chapter 11   Depth of Field 289
  • Chapter 12   Magnifying Devices 291
  • Chapter 13   Retinal Image Size 293
  • Chapter 14   Reflection 295
  • Chapter 15   Aberrations 302

Index **305**

Preface

The goal of this book is to demystify geometrical and visual optics. It is intended to be a concise and learner-friendly resource for clinicians as they study optics for the first time and subsequently prepare for licensing and qualifying examinations. The emphasis is on those optical concepts and problem-solving skills that underlie contemporary clinical eye care and refraction.

The book stresses a vergence approach to geometrical and visual optics. Schematic figures and clinical examples are used throughout the text to engage reader interest. Every effort is made to provide the reader with an intuitive and clinical sense of optics that will allow him or her to effectively care for patients.

To develop competence and facility in geometrical and visual optics, it is necessary to solve problems. Each chapter provides problems of varying complexity, with worked-out solutions given at the end of the book. The reader should make every attempt to solve the problems before resorting to the solutions.

Despite careful review and editing, mathematical errors are bound to occur in a text of this nature. Please send any corrections or comments to the author at *<opticsbook@aol.com>*.

This book grew out of my experiences as an educator and practitioner. Over the years, I have been afforded the opportunity to work with talented colleagues, teach motivated students, and provide care to a diverse spectrum of patients. My colleagues, students, and patients all, in their own ways, motivated this book and for this I am most thankful.

Drs. Raymond Applegate, Ian Bailey, Michael Barris, Lewis Reich, and Alan Riezman read and commented on portions of the manuscript. Their thoughtful input is very much appreciated.

Sally Barhydt, Charissa Baker, Darlene Cooke, and Lester Sheinis, all of McGraw-Hill, and Dr. Norman Haffner, President of the State University of New York, State College of Optometry, provided critical support at various stages of this project. The forbearance and encouragement of Lenge Hong throughout this past year is especially appreciated.

GEOMETRICAL
AND
VISUAL OPTICS

Basic Terms and Concepts

At any given moment, our eyes are inundated by an enormous quantity of electromagnetic radiation. This radiation ranges from short-wavelength gamma and x-ray radiation to longer-wavelength radar and radio waves. *Light* is the portion of the electromagnetic spectrum that is visible (Fig. 1-1).

Electromagnetic radiation is typically specified by its wavelength or frequency. Wavelength and frequency are inversely proportional and related to each other as shown by the following equation:

$$\nu = c/\lambda \; \checkmark$$

where

ν = the frequency of light
c = the speed of light
λ = the wavelength of light

The wavelength of light ranges from about 380 to 700 nanometers (nm).[1] It is emitted in discrete packages of energy referred to as *photons* or *quanta*. The amount of energy in a photon is given by the following relationship:

$$E = h\nu \; \checkmark$$

where

E = the amount of energy per photon
h = Planck's constant

---

[1]One nanometer (nm) is equal to 10^{-9} meters (m).

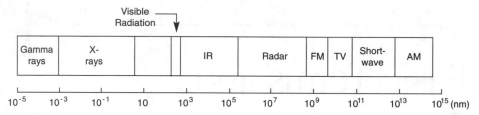

FIGURE 1-1. Light (visible radiation) is a small portion of the electromagnetic spectrum. (*From Schwartz SH*. Visual Perception: A Clinical Orientation. *Copyright 1999. Reprinted by permission of McGraw-Hill, Inc.*)

By substitution, we have:

$$E = \frac{hc}{\lambda}$$

As the wavelength decreases, the amount of energy per photon increases. For this reason, the absorption of short-wavelength radiation by body tissues is typically more damaging than the absorption of longer-wavelength radiation. The development of cataracts and basal cell carcinoma is promoted by exposure to short-wavelength, high-energy ultraviolet radiation.

OBJECTS, LIGHT RAYS, AND PENCILS

We see *objects* because they emit or reflect light, and this light is focused on our retina. A *point source* of light, such as a star, emits waves of light in much the same way that a pebble dropped into a quiet pond of water generates waves of water (Fig. 1-2). Light *rays* are perpendicular to light wavefronts and are represented by arrows.

A bundle of rays is called a *pencil* (Fig. 1-3). The light rays that form a pencil can be diverging, converging, or parallel. A *diverging pencil* is produced by a point source of light, such as a star. When light rays are focused at a point, they create a *converging pencil.* A converging optical system (e.g., a magnifying lens) is required to create converging light. An object located infinitely far away forms a *parallel pencil.*[2]

An *extended object,* such as an arrow, is composed of an infinite number of point sources (Fig. 1-4). Diverging light rays emerge from the point sources.

---

[2]Consider the waves that are created when a pebble is dropped into a quiet pond of water (Fig. 1-2). The wavefronts closest to the source (the pebble) are more curved than the wavefronts further from the source. At very far distances, the wavefronts are flat. Since rays are perpendicular to wavefronts, the rays are parallel to each other.

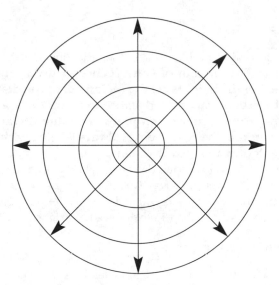

FIGURE 1-2. A point source of light emits concentric waves of light in much the same way a pebble dropped into a quiet pond of water produces waves of water. Light rays, represented by arrows, are orthogonal to the wavefronts.

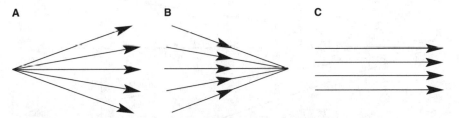

FIGURE 1-3A. A diverging pencil of light rays emerges from a point source. **B.** A converging pencil of light rays is focused at a point. **C.** An object located at infinity produces a parallel pencil of light rays.

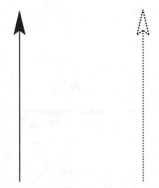

FIGURE 1-4. An extended object, such as an arrow, may be considered to consist of an infinite number of point sources. Each point emits diverging light rays.

VERGENCE

For solving clinical optical problems, it is useful to quantify the convergence or divergence of light. **The amount of convergence or divergence of light rays (i.e., the *vergence* of the light) is (1) the reciprocal of the distance to a point source or (2) the reciprocal of the distance to a point of focus. To arrive at the correct units for vergence—*diopters (D)*—the distance must be in meters. By convention, diverging light is always labeled with a negative sign and converging light with a positive sign.**

Consider Figure 1-5, which shows diverging light rays. At a distance of 10.00 cm from the point source, the vergence is − 10.00 diopters, or − 10.00 D.[3] At distances of 20.00 and 50.00 cm, the vergence is −5.00 and −2.00 D, respectively. The further the distance from the point source, the less the (absolute) magnitude of the divergence.[4]

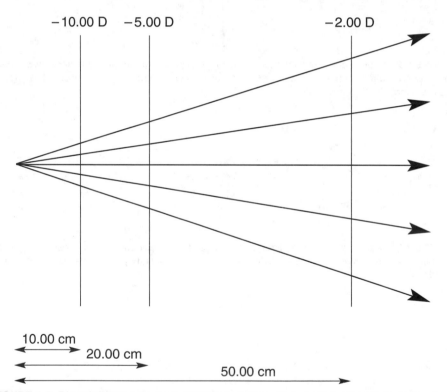

FIGURE 1-5. Diverging light rays have negative vergence. The absolute magnitude of the divergence *decreases* as the distance from the object *increases*.

---

[3]The reciprocal of 0.10 is 10.00.

[4]Returning to Figure 1-2, the wavefronts that are closer to the source are more curved than those further from the source. You can think of the curvature of a wavefront as a measure of vergence—the more curved the wavefront, the greater the vergence. In the extreme case—at an infinite distance from the source—the wavefront is flat (the rays are parallel), and the vergence is zero.

In Figure 1-6, converging light rays are focused at a point. With respect to this point of focus, the vergence at 50.00 cm is +2.00 D. Likewise, at distances of 20.00 and 10.00 cm, the vergence is +5.00 and +10.00 D, respectively. As the distance from the point of focus increases, the magnitude of the convergence decreases.

What is the vergence of parallel light rays? These rays originate from an object at optical infinity; the reciprocal of infinity is zero.[5] Or think of it this way: since the rays are neither diverging nor converging, their vergence is zero.

REFRACTION

When light travels from one transparent material (e.g., air) to a more optically dense transparent material (e.g., water), its velocity decreases. This decrease in velocity can cause light rays to deviate from their original direction, a phenomenon referred to as *refraction*. In Figure 1-7A, a light ray traveling through air

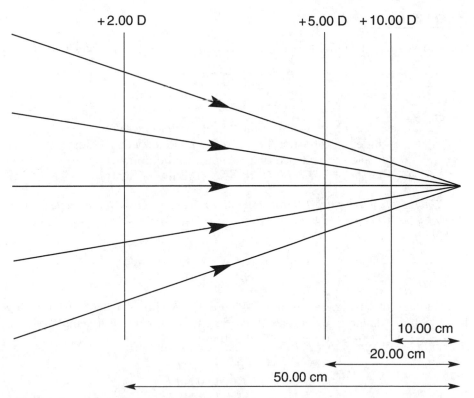

FIGURE 1-6. Converging light rays have positive vergence. As the distance from the point of focus *increases*, the absolute magnitude of the convergence *decreases*.

---

[5]In clinical practice, optical infinity is typically a distance of 20 ft (or 6 m).

strikes the surface of water at an angle of 20.00 degrees. (The angle is measured with respect to the normal course to the surface.) Upon entering water, the light ray deviates, so that it now forms an angle of 14.90 degrees with the normal. That is, the light ray has been refracted.

There are a few rules to remember regarding refraction:

1. Each transparent material (or medium) has an *index of refraction*.[6] Light travels more slowly in media that have high indices of refraction (Table 1-1).

2. When a light ray travels from a material with a low index of refraction (an optically rarefied medium) to one with a higher index of refraction (an optically denser medium), the light ray is refracted *toward* (i.e., bent toward) the normal to the surface (as in Fig. 1-7A). Upon entering a lower index of refraction, the ray is refracted *away* from the normal (Figure 1-7B).

Figure 1-8 shows a light ray traveling from water to air to crown glass. The deviation of the light ray at each of the three surfaces is predictable based upon the above rules.

SNELL'S LAW

Snell's law quantifies the refraction that occurs at a surface. It states that

$$n \sin \theta = n' \sin \theta'$$

Where

n = index of refraction of the *primary* (first) medium
n' = index of refraction of the *secondary* (second) medium
θ = angle of incidence (with respect to the normal)
θ' = angle of refraction (with respect to the normal)

The light ray in Figure 1-9 travels from air to crown glass. If the angle of incidence is 20.00 degrees, what is the angle of refraction?

$$n \sin \theta = n' \sin \theta'$$
$$1.00 \sin 20.00° = 1.52 \sin \theta'$$
$$\theta' = 13.00°$$

Let us look at another example. Figure 1-10A shows a light ray traveling from within a diamond toward air. According to Snell's law, if the angle of incidence is 5.00 degrees, the angle of refraction is

$$n \sin \theta = n' \sin \theta'$$
$$2.42 \sin 5.00° = 1.00 \sin \theta'$$
$$\theta' = 12.18°$$

---

[6]The index of refraction of a material is the ratio of the speed of light in a vacuum to the speed of light in the material.

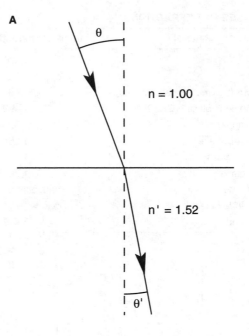

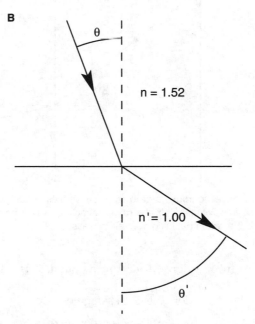

FIGURE 1-7A. A light ray entering a denser medium is refracted *toward* the normal. **B.** A ray entering a rarer medium is refracted *away* from the normal.

TABLE 1-1. SOME INDICES OF REFRACTION

Material	Index of Refraction
Air	1.000
Water	1.333
PMMA (polymethylmethacrylate)	1.49
Ophthalmic plastic (CR39)	1.498
Crown glass	1.523
Polycarbonate	1.586
Barium glass	~ 1.60
Flint glass	~ 1.70
High-index plastics	Variable
High-index glass	Up to > 1.70
Diamond	2.417

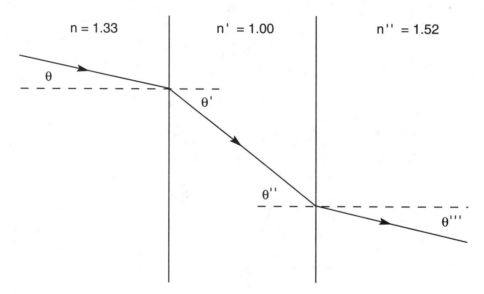

FIGURE 1-8. A light ray traveling from water to air to crown glass undergoes refraction at each surface. When traveling from water to air, the ray is refracted away from the normal, while it is refracted toward the normal when traveling from air to glass.

Since the ray travels from a dense to a rare medium, it is refracted away from the normal.

What if the angle of incidence is 24.41 degrees?

$$2.42 \sin 24.41° = 1.00 \sin \theta'$$
$$\theta' \approx 90.00°$$

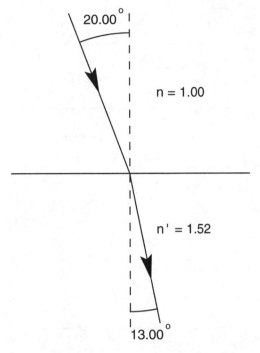

FIGURE 1-9. A light ray that strikes a crown glass surface at an angle of 20.00 degrees has an angle of refraction of 13.00 degrees.

In this case, the refracted ray is parallel to the surface (Fig. 1-10B). When the angle of incidence exceeds 24.41 degrees, the so-called *critical angle*, the light ray undergoes what is called *total internal reflection*—**it does not emerge from the material** (Fig. 1-10C). This is the principle that underlies the *goniolens*, a contact lens–like device that is used to examine the clinically important angle of the eye formed by the cornea and the iris (Fig. 1-11).

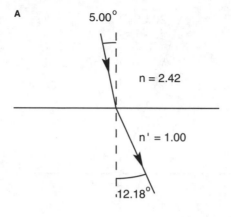

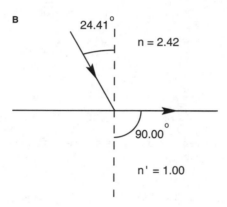

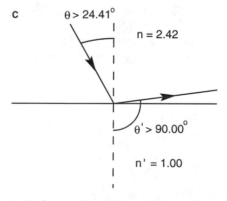

FIGURE 1-10. A light ray travels from a diamond toward air. **A.** For an angle of incidence of 5.00 degrees, the angle of refraction is 12.18 degrees. **B.** If the angle of incidence is 24.41 degrees, the angle of refraction is 90.00 degrees. The refracted ray is parallel to the surface. **C.** When the angle of incidence exceeds the critical angle (24.41 degrees), the light ray undergoes total internal reflection.

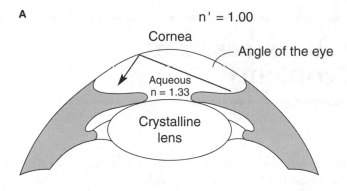

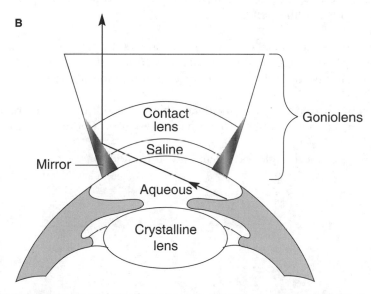

FIGURE 1-11A. A light ray emerging from the angle of the eye undergoes total internal reflection if the angle of incidence (at the cornea) exceeds ~ 49 degrees. (The light ray is traveling from the denser aqueous toward the rarer air.) Total internal reflection prevents the doctor from examining the angle unless he or she uses a device referred to as a *goniolens*. **B.** A goniolens allows visualization of the angle of the eye by reducing total internal reflection. A saline-like fluid is placed between the contact lens that constitutes the front of the goniolens and the cornea. Since the saline and the aqueous humor have about the same index of refraction, total internal reflection is substantially reduced, and the ray emerging from the angle passes out of the eye. It is then reflected by a mirror in the goniolens, thereby allowing examination of the angle. The doctor looks into the mirror and sees a reflection of the structures that constitute the angle. (This diagram is a simplification.)

P Self-Assessment Problems

1. A ray of light emerges from a pond of water at an angle of 45 degrees to the normal. What angle did the incident ray make with the normal?

2. A ray of light is incident upon a pond of water that is 2.0 m deep. If the angle of incidence is 25 degrees, by how many centimeters is the ray deviated as it travels through the pond?

3. A crown glass slab, 75.00 cm thick, is surrounded by air. A ray of light makes an angle of 30 degrees to the normal at the front surface of the slab. At what angle (to the normal) does the ray emerge from the slab?

4. What is the smallest angle of incidence that will result in total internal reflection for a light ray traveling from a high-index glass (index of 1.72) to air?

5. What is the critical angle for a diamond surrounded by water?

Refraction at Spherical Surfaces

2

CONVERGING AND DIVERGING SURFACES

Figure 2-1A shows parallel light rays striking a plane (flat) glass surface. Although there is a change in the index of refraction as the light rays travel from the primary medium (air) to the secondary medium (glass), the angle of incidence is zero and refraction does not occur (Snell's law). The same holds true for a *spherical glass surface*[1] if light rays are directed toward its *center of curvature* (*C*), striking the surface perpendicular to its surface; these light rays are not refracted (Fig. 2-1B).

Now, consider parallel light rays (originating from an object located at infinity) that are incident upon a spherical glass surface (Fig. 2-2). Rays 1, 2, 4, and 5 are each refracted toward the normal to the surface (i.e., the surface's radius of curvature). The amount of refraction, as given by Snell's law, is greater for those rays that have a larger angle of incidence. Hence, ray 1 is refracted more than ray 2, and ray 5 is refracted more than ray 4. Ray 3 is not refracted at all (it is not deviated) because it is normal to the glass surface and has an angle of incidence of zero degrees. This ray travels along the surface's *optical axis*, which connects the center of curvature and the surface's focal points (defined below).

The crown glass surface illustrated in Figure 2-2 *converges* light. Such a surface is often called *positive* or *plus* because it adds positive vergence (i.e., convergence) to rays of light.

Light rays that originate at infinity—traveling from the primary medium (index of *n*) into the secondary medium (index of *n′*)—converge at a point, *F′*, which is defined as the *secondary focal point* of the surface (Fig. 2-2). The distance from the surface apex to the secondary focal point is the *secondary focal*

---

[1] As its name implies, a spherical surface is a section of a sphere. Its radius, also called its *radius of curvature*, is the distance from the surface to the center of curvature.

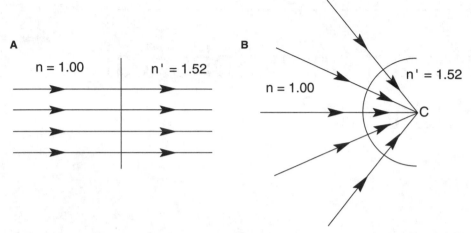

FIGURE 2-1A. Parallel light rays that are incident upon a plane glass surface are not deviated. **B.** Similarly, rays headed toward the center of curvature (*C*) of a spherical glass surface strike the surface orthogonal to its surface and are not deviated. A spherical surface is a section of a sphere. Its radius, which is frequently referred to as its *radius of curvature*, is the distance from the surface to the center of curvature.

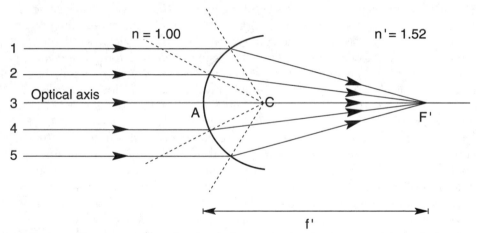

FIGURE 2-2. Parallel light rays that are incident upon a converging spherical glass surface are focused at *F'*, the surface's secondary focal point. The dotted lines are normal to the spherical surface. As the rays travel from air to glass, they are refracted toward the normal. The optical axis connects the center of curvature and the secondary focal point. The distance from the apex of the surface, *A*, to the secondary focal point is the secondary focal length, *f'*. All material to the right of the surface is assumed to be glass.

length, f'. The *refractive power* of the surface[2] (in diopters) is calculated by multiplying the reciprocal of the secondary focal length (in meters) by the index of refraction of the secondary medium (n')—the medium in which the refracted rays exist. This is expressed as

---

[2] The terms *refractive power* and *dioptric power* are used interchangeably.

$$|P| = |n'/f'|$$ If f in 2° media n'

This formula gives us the *absolute* value of the surface's refractive power. For example, if the secondary focal length of the convex surface in Figure 2-2 is 20.00 cm, the surface power is calculated as

$$|P| = |1.52/0.20 \text{ m}|$$

Since the surface converges light, its power must be designated with a plus sign, as indicated below:

$$P = +7.60 \text{ D}$$

The power of an optical system must always be preceded by a plus or minus sign. Converging systems are designated by a plus sign and diverging systems with a minus sign.

Next, consider the crown glass spherical surface in Figure 2-3. Parallel light rays incident upon the denser secondary surface are bent toward the normal. Because of the concave curvature of the glass, the light rays *diverge*. This is a *negative* (or *minus* surface) because it increases the divergence (i.e., negative vergence) of the light rays.

When parallel light rays are refracted by this minus surface, they diverge in the secondary medium (n'), and appear to originate from what we define as the surface's *secondary focal point* (F'). As is the case with a converging surface, the surface power is given by the relationship shown at the top of page 16.

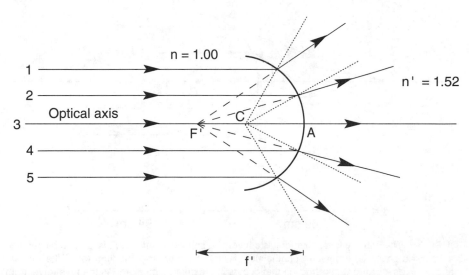

FIGURE 2-3. Parallel rays that are incident upon a diverging spherical glass surface appear to diverge from *F'*, the surface's secondary focal point. Dashed lines connect the refracted rays to *F'*. The dotted lines are orthogonal to the spherical surface. As the rays travel from air to glass, they are refracted toward the normal. All material to the right of the surface is assumed to be glass.

$$|P| = |n'/f'|$$

If the secondary focal point for the spherical surface in Figure 2-3 is 20.00 cm to the left of the surface, then

$$|P| = |1.52/0.20 \text{ m}|$$

Since this is a diverging surface, we must designate its power with a minus sign, as follows:

$$P = -7.60 \text{ D}$$

MORE ON FOCAL POINTS

Let us formally define the secondary focal point of a spherical surface. When parallel light rays travel from the *primary medium to the secondary medium*, the secondary focal point is (1) the point to which the light converges (Fig. 2-2) or (2) the point from which the light appears to diverge (Fig. 2-3). **The secondary**

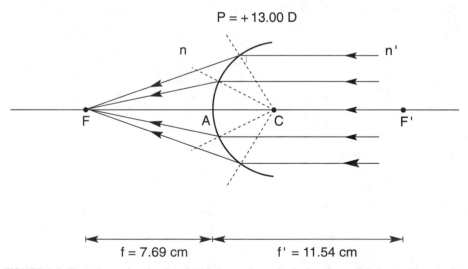

FIGURE 2-4. The primary focal point of this converging spherical surface, *F*, is located by sending rays from the secondary medium (ophthalmic plastic) to the primary medium (air). The primary focal point is associated with refraction that occurs in the primary medium. As the rays travel from plastic to air, they are refracted away from the normal. The surface has a power of +13.00 D, as indicated at the top of the surface. All material to the right of the surface is assumed to be plastic.

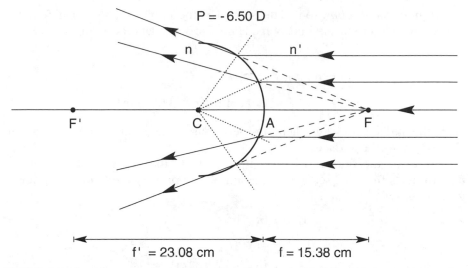

FIGURE 2-5. The primary focal point of this diverging spherical surface, *F*, is located by sending rays from the secondary medium (ophthalmic plastic) to the primary medium (air). The primary focal point is associated with refraction that occurs in the primary medium. As the rays travel from plastic to air, they are refracted away from the normal. The surface has a power of –6.50 D, as indicated at the top of the surface. All material to the right of the surface is assumed to be plastic.

focal point is associated with the refraction that occurs as light enters the secondary medium.

A refracting surface also has a *primary focal point* (*F*), which is located by reversing the direction of the light rays. When parallel light travels from the *secondary medium to the primary medium*, the primary focal point is (1) the point to which the light converges or (2) the point from which the light appears to diverge. **The primary focal point is associated with the refraction that occurs as light enters the primary medium.** *

Where is the primary focal point for the converging surface in Figure 2-4? To locate *F*, we reverse the direction of the light rays so that they travel from the secondary to the primary medium (rather than from the primary to secondary medium, as we have discussed up to now). These rays are bent away from the normal as they enter the primary medium and converge at the primary focal point *F*. The distance from the apex of the surface to the primary focal point is the *primary focal length (f)*.

The location of the primary focal point for a *diverging* surface is illustrated in Figure 2-5. The light rays travel in a reverse direction, from the secondary medium to the primary medium. Refraction occurs as the rays enter the primary medium; the focal point associated with this refraction is *F*.

Let us solve a problem. *Assume that the spherical surface in Figure 2-4 is made of ophthalmic plastic and has a refractive power of +13.00 D. Locate the secondary and primary focal points.* To find the secondary focal point, we send light from the primary medium to the secondary medium. The secondary focal length is

$$|P| = |n'/f'|$$

$$|+13.00\ D| = |1.50/f'|$$

$$|f'| = |0.1154\ m|\ \text{or}\ |11.54\ cm|$$

Since the surface converges light, the secondary focal point is located 11.54 cm to the right of the surface.

To locate the primary focal point, we reverse the direction of the light so that it travels from the secondary medium to the primary medium. The primary focal length is

$$|P| = |n/f|$$

$$|+13.00\ D| = |1.00/f|$$

$$|f| = |0.0769\ m|\ \text{or}\ |7.69\ cm|$$

The primary focal point for this converging system is located 7.69 cm to the left of the surface. The focal distances are labeled in Figure 2-4.

Assume that the spherical surface in Figure 2-5 is made of plastic and has a power of −6.50 D. Locate the secondary and primary focal points. The secondary focal point is associated with the refraction that occurs as light traveled from the primary to secondary medium. The secondary focal length is

$$|P| = |n'/f'|$$

$$|-6.50\ D| = |1.50/f'|$$

$$|f'| = |0.2308\ m|\ \text{or}\ |23.08\ cm|$$

Since the surface diverges light, the secondary focal point is located 23.08 cm to the left of the surface (Fig. 2-5).

The primary focal point is associated with the refraction that occurs when light travels from the secondary to primary medium. The primary focal length is

$$|P| = |n/f|$$

$$|-6.50\ D| = |1.00/f|$$

$$|f| = |0.1538\ m|\ \text{or}\ |15.38\ cm|$$

The primary focal point for this diverging system is located 15.38 cm to the right of the surface.

REFRACTING POWER AND FOCAL LENGTHS

A refracting surface has the same *power* regardless of whether the light rays travel from the primary to secondary medium or vice versa. As Figures 2-4 and

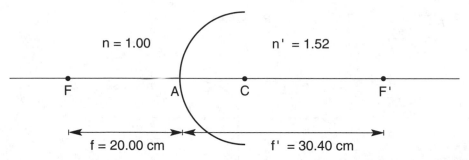

FIGURE 2-6 The primary focal length (*f*) of a glass surface is not equal to the secondary focal length of the surface (*f'*). All distances are measured from the apex of the surface, which is designated by the vertical line. All material to the right of the surface is assumed to be glass.

2-5 illustrate, however, the primary focal length of a spherical refracting surface is *not* equal to the secondary focal length.

Let us look at another example. *Consider a positive crown glass spherical surface with a secondary focal length of 30.40 cm (Fig. 2-6). What is the power of the surface? What is its primary focal length?* The power is calculated as

$$|P| = |n'/f'|$$
$$|P| = |1.52/0.304 \text{ m}|$$
$$|P| = |5.00 \text{ D}|$$

Since the surface is positive,

$$P = +5.00 \text{ D}$$

For the primary focal length,

$$|P| = |n/f|$$
$$|5.00 \text{ D}| = |1.00/f|$$
$$|f| = |0.20 \text{ m}| \text{ or } |20.00 \text{ cm}|$$

The secondary focal point of this +5.00 D surface is located 30.40 cm to the right of the surface, while the primary focal point is located 20.00 cm to the left of the surface.

ANOTHER WAY TO CALCULATE POWER

By definition, a spherical surface is derived from a sphere. The radius of the sphere can be used to calculate the refracting power with the relationship shown at the top of page 21.[3]

---

[3] This relationship is derived in Chapter 15.

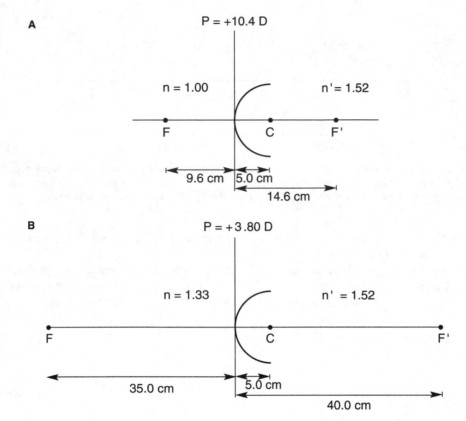

A

P = +10.4 D

n = 1.00   n' = 1.52

F   C   F'

9.6 cm | 5.0 cm

14.6 cm

B

P = +3.80 D

n = 1.33   n' = 1.52

F   C   F'

35.0 cm   5.0 cm

40.0 cm

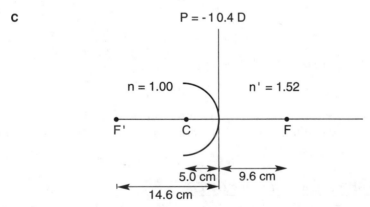

C

P = -10.4 D

n = 1.00   n' = 1.52

F'   C   F

5.0 cm | 9.6 cm

14.6 cm

FIGURE 2-7A. A converging crown glass surface, with a radius of curvature of 5.0 cm, is situated in air. **B.** When the surface in **A** is placed in water, its refractive power is less and its focal lengths are longer. **C.** A diverging crown glass surface, with a radius of curvature of 5.0 cm, is situated in air. All distances in this figure are measured from the apices of the surfaces, which are indicated by the vertical lines. Refractive powers are given at the top of each surface. All material to the right of the surface is assumed to be glass. (The reader should calculate the focal lengths for the surfaces in this figure to confirm the labeled values.)

$$|P| = \left| \frac{n' - n}{r} \right|$$

The *radius of curvature* (*r*)—the distance from the surface to its center of curvature—must be in meters. This equation tells us that the more curved a surface (or the shorter its radius), the greater its power.

We can use this relationship to determine the refractive power of the crown glass spherical surface in Figure 2-7A. This surface has a radius of curvature of 5.00 cm. Its power is calculated as follows:

$$|P| = \left| \frac{n' - n}{r} \right|$$

$$|P| = \left| \frac{1.52 - 1.00}{0.05 \text{ m}} \right|$$

Since the surface is converging, we designate its power with a positive sign:

$$P = +10.40 \text{ D}$$

What is the power of this same glass surface when it is immersed in water (Fig. 2-7B)?

$$|P| = \left| \frac{n' - n}{r} \right|$$

$$|P| = \left| \frac{1.52 - 1.33}{0.05 \text{ m}} \right|$$

We designate the power of this converging lens with a positive sign:

$$P = +3.80 \text{ D}$$

Note that as the indices of the primary and secondary media become more similar, there is a *reduction* in the surface's refractive power and a consequent *increase* in the primary and secondary focal lengths.[4]

Now, let us calculate the power of the diverging crown glass surface in Figure 2-7C, which has a radius of curvature of 5.00 cm.

$$|P| = \left| \frac{n' - n}{r} \right|$$

$$|P| = \left| \frac{1.52 - 1.00}{0.05 \text{ m}} \right|$$

$$P = -10.40 \text{ D}$$

---

[4] The reader should confirm that the focal lengths given in Figure 2-7 are correct.

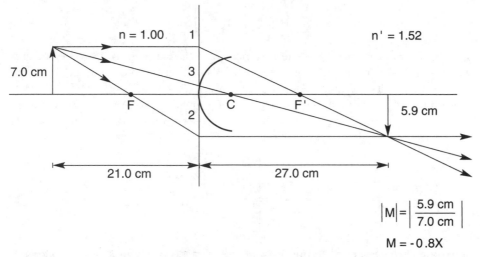

$$|M| = \left| \frac{5.9 \text{ cm}}{7.0 \text{ cm}} \right|$$

$$M = -0.8X$$

FIGURE 2-8. Ray tracing can be used to locate an image and determine its size. When an object is outside of the primary focal length of a converging surface, the image is real, inverted, and minified. All distances are measured from the plane of the surface's apex (*A*), which is designated by the vertical line. The magnification (*M*) produced by the surface is the ratio of the image height to the object height. Since the image is inverted, the magnification is designated with a minus sign. All material to the right of the surface is assumed to be glass.

Note that this diverging surface has the same primary and secondary focal lengths (absolute values) as the converging surface in Figure 2-7A.

REAL IMAGES

Figure 2-8 shows an object that is located to the left of a converging crown glass spherical surface.[5] Light rays diverge from each point on the object. Three specific rays, which originate from the tip of the arrow and travel from the primary to the secondary index, allow us to locate the image of the arrow's tip.[6]

Ray 1 originates from the object, travels parallel to the optical axis in the primary index, and after refraction is deviated through *F'*. Passing though *F*, ray 2 is refracted at the surface so that it is parallel to the optical axis in the secondary medium. Since ray 3 is perpendicular to the spherical surface (it is headed toward the surface's center of curvature), it is not deviated. The point where all three rays intersect is the *image* of the arrow's tip. We have traced only three rays, but all rays that originate from the tip of the arrow (there are an infinite number of such rays) are focused here. By definition, objects and images are *conjugate* with each other.

---

[5] Although we have been using the terms primary medium and secondary medium, we have not explicitly defined these terms. It is within the primary medium that the object is typically located. Light rays emerging from the object travel toward the secondary medium.
[6] All distances are measured from the apex of the surface, which is indicated by a vertical line. Refraction is assumed to occur in this plane. All material to the right of this plane is the secondary medium (glass).

Because the diagram is drawn to scale, we can locate the image with respect to the surface. By comparing the sizes of the object and image (using a ruler), we can also determine the *magnification* produced by the surface. Figure 2-8 and the subsequent ray diagram in this chapter are drawn to scale, with the object and image distances and sizes given, along with the magnification.

Note that the arrow is *inverted*. An inverted image is designated by a minus sign preceding the magnification.

The image is a *real* image because it is formed by converging light rays. If a screen is placed in the plane of the image, the arrow will be focused on this screen.

VIRTUAL IMAGES

Consider the arrow that is imaged by the diverging crown glass spherical surface in Figure 2-9. Ray 1 originates parallel to the optical axis in the primary medium and is diverged at the surface so that it appears to emerge from F'. Ray 2 is headed toward F and is refracted so that it is parallel to the optical axis in

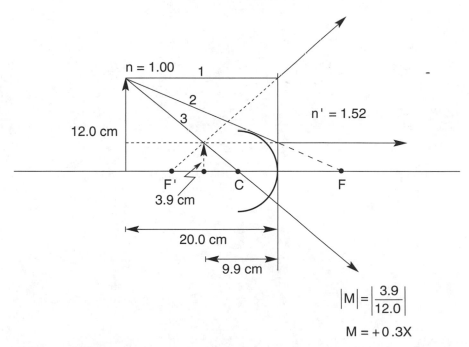

$$|M| = \left| \frac{3.9}{12.0} \right|$$

$$M = +0.3X$$

FIGURE 2-9. A diverging surface produces a virtual image (the dashed arrow) that is erect and minified. All distances are measured from the plane of the surface's apex (*A*), which is indicated by the vertical line. (For illustrative purposes, the object is drawn larger than the surface.) Since the image is erect, its magnification is designated with a positive sign. All material to the right of the surface is assumed to be glass.

the secondary medium. Finally, ray 3 travels through the glass surface's center of curvature, striking the surface perpendicular to its surface.

The light rays that *exist* in the secondary medium *appear* to emerge from a single point located in the primary medium. *Dashed lines* connect the diverging light rays in the secondary medium to the image from which they appear to come. All rays that are emitted from the arrow's tip *appear* to emerge from this image. Since the rays appear to come from the image and are not actually focused in the plane of the image (except for ray 3, which is an exception), the image is *virtual.* Dashed lines are used to draw a virtual image.

Virtual images are formed by diverging light rays. A virtual image cannot be focused on a screen—it is not formed by converging light rays. The image is, however, visible. If you could place your eye into the glass material and view the diverging light rays, you would see a virtual image of the arrow, not the arrow itself. Note that the arrow is erect and that its magnification is designated by a plus sign.

P | Self-Assessment Problems

1. (a) Is the crown glass spherical surface drawn below converging or diverging? (b) What is its power if its radius of curvature is 15.00 mm? (c) Locate and label *F* and *F'*.

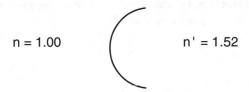

n = 1.00   n' = 1.52

2. For the crown glass spherical surface below, answer the questions in Problem 1. The radius of curvature is 200.00 mm.

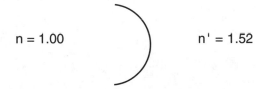

n = 1.00   n' = 1.52

3. Label each of the following refracting surfaces as plus or minus.

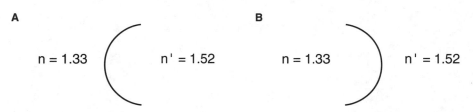

A

n = 1.33   n' = 1.52

B

n = 1.33   n' = 1.52

C

n = 1.72   n' = 1.00

D

n = 1.00   n' = 1.72

4. An object, 3.0 cm in height, is located in air. It is 9.0 cm in front of a −10.00 D crown glass surface. (a) On a diagram drawn to scale, label the primary and secondary focal points and radius of curvature. (b) Use ray tracing to determine the image distance from the apex of the surface and the size of the image. (c) What is the magnification of the image? (d) Is the image erect or inverted? Is it real or virtual? Explain.

5. Answer the questions in Problem 4 for a 2.0 cm-high object located 20 cm in front of a + 10.00 D crown glass surface.

6. A rock sits on the bottom of a pond 3.0 m deep. (a) Does the rock appear to be 3.0 m from the upper surface of the pond? Explain with a diagram. (b) Is the image of the rock real or virtual?

The Vergence Relationship

3

BASIC CONCEPTS

As we learned in the previous chapter, ray diagrams can be used to determine the location and size of an image. The *vergence relationship*, sometimes referred to as the *paraxial relationship*, provides a convenient alternative method to locate images and to determine the magnification produced by an optical system.

All real objects emit diverging bundles of light rays. The vergence of these light rays—negative vergence—can be quantified as described in Chapter 1. A spherical refracting element, such as a spherical refracting surface or lens, changes the vergence of the light rays that are incident upon it. You will find it helpful to think of a spherical refracting surface as a *vergence changer*. After their vergence has been changed, the rays form an image. These concepts are represented in the vergence relationship, as follows[1]:

$$\text{vergence incident on surface} + \text{refractive power of surface}$$
$$= \text{vergence leaving surface}$$

or

$$\text{object vergence} + \text{surface power} = \text{image vergence}$$

---

[1] This relationship applies only to paraxial rays—those light rays that are in relatively close proximity to the optical axis of the surface. For these rays, the angle of incidence, θ (in radians), approximates $\sin \theta$. Most basic optical problems can be solved by assuming that the rays are paraxial. See Chapter 15 for a derivation of the paraxial equation.

Designating the object vergence as L, the surface power as P, and the image vergence as L', we have[2]

$$L + P = L'$$
or

$$L' = L + P$$

The sign of the image vergence tells us whet   her the image is real or virtual. If the rays are converging (i.e., positive vergence), the image is real. When the rays are diverging (negative vergence), the image is virtual.

MORE ON VERGENCE

As we learned in Chapter 1, the amount of light ray vergence (either divergence or convergence) is (1) the reciprocal of the distance to a point source or (2) the reciprocal of the distance to a point of focus. To arrive at the correct units of vergence—*diopters* (D)—the distance must be in meters.

The vergence of light rays emitted from an object that is located in air is the reciprocal of the distance to the object. This distance is designated as l. The absolute value of the object vergence is given by

$$|L| = |1.00/l| \qquad \text{1.00 AIR or n}$$

For the object in Figure 3-1A, the vergence is

$$|L| = |1.00/0.33 \text{ m}|$$

Since the light rays are diverging, the object vergence is designated with a minus sign, thus:

$$L = -3.03 \text{ D}$$

When the object is located in a medium other than air, the medium's index of refraction influences the vergence. For an object located in a medium n, the vergence is given by the following relationship:

$$|L| = |n/l|$$

What is the vergence for the object in Figure 3-1B that is located in water rather than air?

---

[2] Unfortunately, a plethora of symbols are used to represent object vergence and image vergence. For example, U is sometimes used to represent object vergence and V to represent image vergence. Do not let this confuse you. Just think in terms of object vergence and image vergence rather than memorizing symbols.

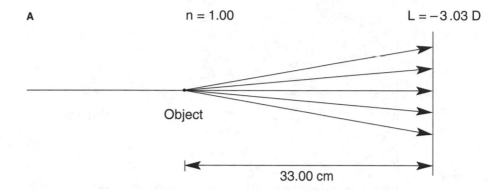

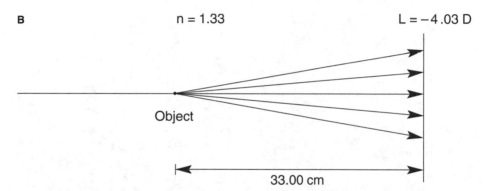

FIGURE 3-1. Object vergence is influenced by the medium in which the light rays exist. The object vergence is greater when the object is located in water than when it is located in air.

$$|L| = |n/l|$$
$$|L| = |1.33/0.33 \text{ m}|$$

Since the rays are diverging, we have

$$L = -4.03 \text{ D}$$

Alternatively, we can place a factor of 100 in the numerator and keep the distance in centimeters, thus[3]

$$|L| = |(100)(1.33)/33.00 \text{ cm}|$$
$$L = -4.03 \text{ D}$$

---

[3] If the distance were in millimeters, we could enter a factor of 1000 in the numerator and keep the distance in millimeters (rather than converting to meters).

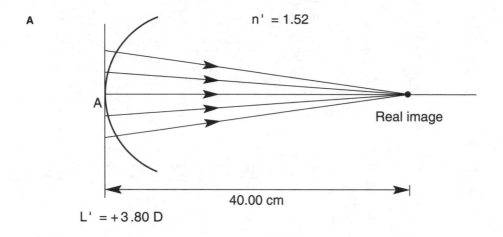

A

n' = 1.52

A

Real image

40.00 cm

L' = +3.80 D

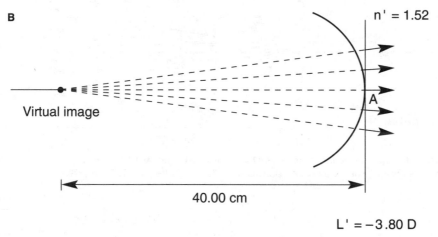

B

n' = 1.52

Virtual image

A

40.00 cm

L' = −3.80 D

FIGURE 3-2A. The vergence for this real image is +3.80 D, as indicated at the bottom of the surface. **B.** The vergence for this virtual image is −3.80 D, as indicated at the bottom of the surface. Recall that for spherical surfaces, refraction is assumed to occur in the plane of the surface's apex (*A*); all distances are measured from this plane.

How do we calculate the vergence of the light rays that form an image? Consider the real image formed by the converging light rays in Figure 3-2A. The image is formed at a distance of 40.00 cm from the refracting surface, and the light rays that form this image exist in crown glass. The image vergence is given by

$$L' = |n'/l'|$$

where

l' = the distance from the refracting surface to the image[4]
n' = the index of the medium in which the rays that form
the image are located (i.e., secondary medium)

For the image in Figure 3-2A, the image vergence is calculated as

$$|L'| = |n'/l'|$$
$$|L'| = |(1.52)(100)/40.00 \text{ cm}|$$

Since the rays that form the real image are converging, the vergence is designated with a plus sign:

$$L' = +3.80 \text{ D}$$

Next, let us determine the vergence for the virtual image in Figure 3-2B. The key is to recognize that the rays forming the image exist in the secondary medium, glass. Therefore, the image vergence is calculated as

$$|L'| = |n'/l'|$$
$$|L'| = |(1.52)(100)/40.00 \text{ cm}|$$

The vergence must be designated with a minus sign since the rays that form the image are diverging:

$$L' = -3.80 \text{ D}$$

SIGN CONVENTIONS

Up to now, we have calculated the absolute value of the vergence and then designated its sign. We have used this approach because it reinforces the important concept of vergence. For convenience, however, we can use a linear sign convention to designate distances as plus or minus and then use these distances to calculate the sign of the vergence.

In this text, we use a sign convention with the following rules: (1) light is assumed to travel from the left to the right, (2) object and image distances are measured *from* the refracting or lens surface, (3) object and image heights are measured *from* the optical axis, (3) distances to the left of the surface are designated as negative and those to the right as positive, and (4) heights above the optical axis are designated as positive and those below the optical axis as negative (Fig. 3-3).

---

[4] As is the case for vergence, all sorts of symbols are used to represent object and image distances. Do not let these confuse you. For example, u is sometimes used to represent object distance and v to represent image distance. The concepts are important, not the symbols!

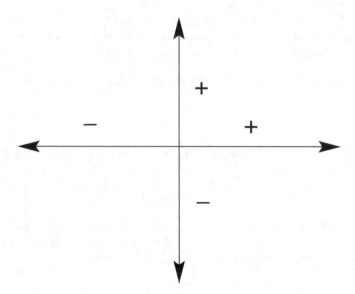

FIGURE 3-3. According to the linear sign convention used in this book, light is assumed to travel from left to right.

Let us use this sign convention to calculate the vergence for the object in Fig. 3-1A. Since the object is located to the left of the surface, the linear distance is −33.00 cm. We use the following relationship to determine the object vergence:

$$L = n/l$$
$$L = (1.00)(100)/-33.00 \text{ cm} = -3.03 \text{ D}$$

For the real image in Figure 3-2A, we have an image distance of +40.00 cm. The image vergence is

$$L' = n'/l'$$
$$L' = (1.52)(100)/+40.00 \text{ cm} = +3.80 \text{ D}$$

And for the virtual image in Fig. 3-2B, which is located 40.00 cm to the left of the surface, the image vergence is

$$L' = n'/l'$$
$$L' = (1.52)(100)/-40.00 \text{ cm} = -3.80 \text{ D}$$

Sample Problems

Converging Surface

An object is located 50.00 cm in front of a +5.00 D spherical crown glass surface. How far is the image from the apex of the surface? Is the image real or virtual? Is it erect or virtual? If the object is 3.00 cm in height, what is the height of the image?

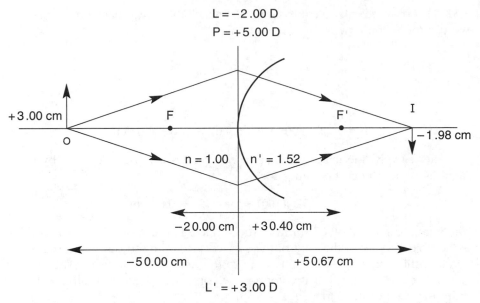

FIGURE 3-4. An object, O, located beyond the primary focal point of a converging surface, forms a real image, I. The rays shown emerge from the base of the object, at the point where it intersects the optical axis. Object vergence and surface power are given above the surface, and image vergence is given below the surface; we will follow this convention throughout this book. *This diagram and others in this chapter are not drawn to scale.*

First, draw a diagram (Fig. 3-4). The object vergence at the refracting surface is

$$L = n/l$$
$$L = 1/-0.50 \text{ m} = -2.00 \text{ D}$$

or

$$L = 100/-50.00 \text{ cm} = -2.00 \text{ D}$$

Light, with a vergence of −2.00 D, is incident upon a surface whose power is +5.00 D. What is the vergence of the light rays after they are refracted? According to the paraxial relationship, the vergence of the light rays that form the image is the sum of the incident vergence and the surface power:

$$L' = L + P$$
$$L' = -2.00 \text{ D} + (+5.00 \text{ D}) = +3.00 \text{ D}$$

Since converging light rays form the image, it is real. Where is it located? The rays that form the image have an image vergence of +3.00 D. **These rays exist in the secondary medium** (glass), which has an index of refraction of

1.52. Therefore, to calculate the distance at which these the image rays converge, we use the secondary index of refraction:

$$L' = n'/l'$$

or

$$l' = n'/L'$$
$$l' = 1.52/+3.00 \text{ D} = +0.5067 \text{ m, or } +50.67 \text{ cm}$$

Alternatively, the image distance in centimeters may be calculated by placing a factor of 100 in the numerator[5]:

$$l' = (1.52\ )(100)/+3.00 \text{ D} = +50.67 \text{ cm}$$

The image is located 50.67 cm from the surface. Is it in front of the surface (as is the object) or or to the right of the surface? According to our linear sign convention, this image is located 50.67 cm to the right of the surface. (This makes sense, because an image that is formed by converging light rays must be located to the right of the surface.)

It is helpful to visualize the light rays in terms of their vergence. In the current example, diverging light rays (−2.00 D) are incident upon a converging surface (+5.00 D). Upon refraction they converge (+3.00 D) to form a real image.

The *lateral magnification* (M_L) produced by the optical system—the ratio of the image size to the object size—is equal to the ratio of the object vergence to the image vergence[6]:

$$M_L = \text{image size/object size} = \text{object vergence/image vergence} = L/L'$$

or simply

$$\boldsymbol{M_L = L/L'}$$

In our sample problem, we have

$$M_L = -2.00 \text{ D}/+3.00 \text{ D} = -0.66X$$

The negative sign tells us that the image is inverted. Since the object height is 3.00 cm, the image height is

$$(-0.66)(3.00 \text{ cm}) = -1.98 \text{ cm}$$

---

[5] If a factor of 1000 is placed in the numerator, the calculated distance would be in millimeters.

[6] Lateral magnification is sometimes called *transverse magnification* or *linear magnification.*

Location of Focal Points

Using the linear sign convention, locate the primary and secondary focal points of the surface in Figure 3-4.

In using the linear sign convention, it is straightforward to locate the secondary focal point:

$$P = n'/f'$$
$$+5.00 \text{ D} = (1.00)(1.52)/f'$$
$$f' = +30.40 \text{ cm}$$

The secondary focal point is 30.40cm to the right of the converging surface.

Now let us try to locate the primary focal point while using the linear sign convention:

$$P = n/f$$
$$+5.00 \text{ D} = (1.00)(1.00)/f$$
$$f = +20.00 \text{ cm}$$

This is not correct! We know that the primary focal point of a converging system is located to the left of the surface, not to the right as indicated by the plus sign in the above answer. To locate the primary focal point, we reverse the direction of light so that it travels from right to left (refer back to Fig. 2-4), not left to right, as it must for the linear sign convention. We can use the linear sign convention if we compensate for this incorrect assumption. This is done by placing a minus sign (a "fudge factor") in front of the relationship that is used to locate the primary focal point:

$$\boldsymbol{P = -n/f}$$

For the lens in Figure 3-4:

$$P = -n/f$$
$$+5.00 \text{ D} = -(1.00)(1.00)/f$$
$$f = -20.00 \text{ cm}$$

The primary focal point is located 20.00 cm to the left of the surface.

Diverging Surface

An object 15.00 cm in height is located 33.00 cm in front of a spherical crown glass surface that has a power of −10.00 D. Locate the image and give its magnification. Is the image real or virtual? Is it erect or inverted?

First, draw a diagram. From Snell's law, we know that the diverging rays emitted by the object are further diverged by the surface (Fig. 3-5). Therefore,

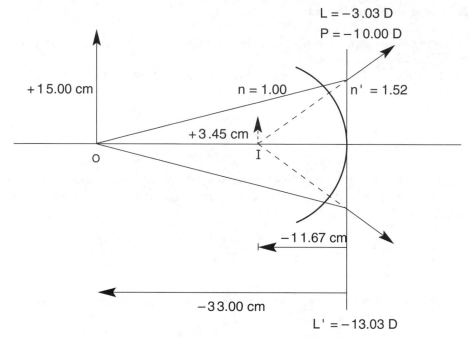

FIGURE 3-5. A negative surface produces a virtual image, *I*.

before we do any calculations we know that the image is: (1) virtual (because it is formed by diverging rays), (2) on the same side of the surface as the object (because the rays that form it appear to diverge from this side of the lens), and (3) closer to the surface than the object (because the divergence has been increased).

To use the vergence relationship, we must first determine the object vergence. Since the object rays exist in air, the object vergence is

$$L = n/l$$
$$L = 100/{-33.00} \text{ cm} = -3.03 \text{ D}$$

This -3.03 D of vergence is incident upon a surface whose power is -10.00 D, resulting in an image vergence of -13.03 D. Or, stated another way,

$$L' = L + P$$
$$L' = -3.03 \text{ D} + -10.00 \text{ D} = -13.03 \text{ D}$$

Because the vergence is negative, the image must be virtual. The refracted image rays exist in glass; therefore, to determine the image distance, we use the index of refraction of crown glass (the secondary medium):

$$L' = n'/l'$$

or

$$l' = n'/L'$$
$$l' = (1.52)(100)/-13.03 \text{ D} = -11.67 \text{ cm}$$

The image is located 11.67 cm to the left of the surface.

The magnification produced by the surface is given by the ratio of the object vergence to the image vergence:

$$M_L = L/L'$$
$$M_L = -3.03D/-13.03 \text{ D} = +0.23X$$

The positive magnification confirms that the image is erect. Since the magnification is less than one, the image is minified. The image size is:

$$(+15.00 \text{ cm})(+0.23) = +3.45 \text{ cm}$$

Locating the Object When Given the Image Location

A virtual image is located 12.00 cm in front of a 5.00 D crown glass diverging spherical surface situated in air. The image is 4.00 cm in height. Locate the object and give its height.

First, draw a diagram that shows a diverging surface forming a virtual image (Fig. 3-6). The figure shows us that diverging light rays form the virtual image and that these rays diverge more than those emitted by the object. The rays that form the image (i.e., the refracted rays) exist in glass. Since the virtual image is to the left of the surface, the image distance is designated with a minus sign. Thus, the image vergence is

$$L' = n'/l'$$
$$L' = (100) \ (1.52)/ -12.00 \text{ cm} = -12.67 \text{ D}$$

The object vergence is given by the paraxial relationship

$$L' = L + P$$
$$-12.67 \text{ D} = L + -5.00 \text{ D}$$
$$L = -7.67 \text{ D}$$

The light rays that emerge from the *object* have a vergence of −7.67 D. These light rays exist in air ($n = 1.00$). The object distance is therefore

$$L = n/l$$
$$l = n/L$$
$$l = (100)(1.00)/-7.67 \text{ D}$$
$$l = -13.04 \text{ cm}$$

The object is on the same side of the surface as the image (both are to the left of the surface) but further from the surface than the image. This is consistent with Figure 3-6.

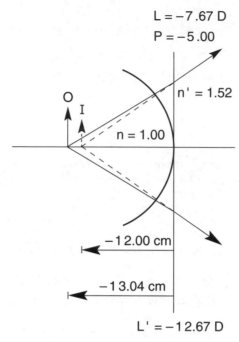

FIGURE 3-6. Given the location of the image, the vergence relationship can be used to locate the object.

The lateral magnification is

$$M_L = L/L'$$
$$M_L = -7.67 \text{ D}/-12.67 \text{ D} = +0.61X$$

Therefore, the object and image have the same orientation, and the image is smaller than the object. The object size is calculated as

$$+4.00 \text{ cm} = (+0.61)(\text{object height})$$
$$\text{object height} = +6.56 \text{ cm}$$

Surface with No Power

A quarter is located at the bottom of an aquarium 38.00 cm from the surface of the water. In looking down into the aquarium, how far does the quarter appear to be from the surface? Is it magnified or minified?

In this problem, light travels upward—not from left to right. This is a bit tricky, because we cannot rely on linear sign conventions. But we can solve the problem if we keep in mind the meaning of negative and positive vergence. The object is real and emits diverging light rays that exist in water, the primary medium (Fig. 3-7). The object vergence is

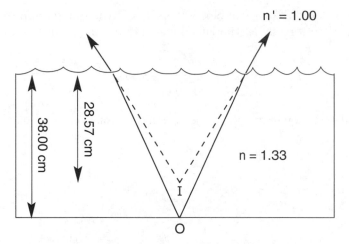

FIGURE 3-7. An object located at the bottom of an aquarium appears to be closer to the surface than it actually is. On looking into the aquarium from above, the viewer sees a virtual image of the coin. The surface refracts light even though it has a dioptric power of zero.

$$|L| = |n/l|$$
$$|L| = |(100)(1.33)/38.00 \text{ cm}|$$

Since the object rays are diverging, the object vergence is as follows:

$$L = -3.50 \text{ D}$$

To determine the image vergence, we use the vergence relationship. The refracting surface is flat and has an infinite radius of curvature; therefore, it has no dioptric power.[7]

$$L' = L + P$$
$$L' = -3.50 \text{ D} + 0.00 \text{ D}$$
$$L' = -3.50 \text{ D}$$

The negative image vergence tells us that the image is virtual. Since diverging rays form the image, it must be located on the same side of the refracting surface as the object. The rays coming from the image exist in air (Fig. 3-7). The image distance is, therefore, calculated as follows:

$$|L'| = |n'/L'|$$
$$|l'| = |(100)(1.00)/-3.50 \text{ D}|$$
$$|l'| = |28.57 \text{ cm}|$$

---

[7]Although the flat surface refracts light, it has no dioptric power—its power is zero diopters.

The image is located 28.57 cm below the surface. The quarter appears closer to the surface than it really is. The lateral magnification is calculated as follows:

$$M_L = L/L'$$
$$M_L = -3.50\ D/-3.50\ D$$
$$M_L = +1.00X$$

The *image* of the quarter is the same size and orientation as a quarter itself.[8]

---

[8] Although the image of the quarter is the same size as the quarter, it appears larger because it is closer to the surface. This is referred to as angular magnification (discussed in Chap. 12).

P Self-Assessment Problems

1. A crown glass spherical surface has a power of −10.00 D. (a) What is the surface's radius of curvature? (b) What is the secondary focal length? (c) What is the primary focal length?

2. A plastic spherical surface has a power of +20.00 D. (a) What is the surface's radius of curvature? (b) What is the secondary focal length? (c) What is the primary focal length?

3. A crown glass spherical surface has a radius of curvature of +15.00 cm. (a) What is the refractive power of the surface? (b) What is the secondary focal length? (c) What is the primary focal length?

4. A polycarbonate spherical surface has a radius of curvature of −125.00 mm. What is the refractive power of the surface?

5. An object 6.00 mm in height is located 20.00 cm from a crown glass spherical surface whose power is −10.00 D. (a) Using the vergence relationship, locate the image and determine its size. (b) Is the image real or virtual? (c) Is the image erect or inverted?

6. An object 10.00 mm in height is located 20.00 cm from a crown glass spherical surface whose power is +10.00 D. (a) Using the vergence relationship, locate the image and determine its size. (b) Is the image real or virtual? (c) Is the image erect or inverted?

7. Answer the questions in Problem 6 if the object is located 5.00 cm from the surface.

8. A virtual image is located 5.00 cm from a +15.00 D crown glass spherical surface. How far is the object from the surface?

9. A real image is located 20.00 cm from a +15.00 D crown glass spherical surface. How far is the object from the surface?

P

10. A rock sits on the bottom of a pond of water that is 3.00 m deep. How far does the rock appear to be from the surface of the pond?

11. The pupil is located 3.60 mm from the cornea. Assume that the cornea has a radius of curvature of 7.80 mm and the aqueous humor has an index of refraction of 1.333. How far does the pupil appear to be from the cornea?

12. If the diameter of the pupil in Problem 11 is 4.00 mm, what does the diameter appear to be?

Thin Lenses

$$4$$

An ophthalmic lens is made up of two surfaces (Fig. 4-1). Each surface of the lens refracts light (Fig. 4-2A). The lens has a finite thickness, and this thickness contributes to its refractive power. In certain instances, however, we can ignore the thickness of the lens[1] and assume that all refraction occurs in a single plane. Such a lens is referred to as a *thin lens*. The total refractive power of a thin lens is the sum of the powers of the two refracting surfaces, as given by the following relationship:

$$P_T = P_1 + P_2$$

where

P_T = the total power of the thin lens
P_1 = the power of the front surface of the lens
P_2 = the power of the back surface of the lens

The powers of the surfaces are given by:

$$P_1 = \frac{n' - n}{r}$$

$$P_2 = \frac{n - n'}{r}$$

As illustrated in Figure 4-2B, thin lenses are represented as vertical lines. In essence, a thin lens is formed by collapsing the front and back surfaces onto a single plane and assuming that all refraction occurs at this plane.

FOCAL POINTS

The primary (F) and secondary (F') focal points for a thin lens are located in the same manner as for a spherical refracting surface (Chap. 2). When parallel

---

[1] The effect of lens thickness is discussed in Chapters 5 and 6.

Plus lenses

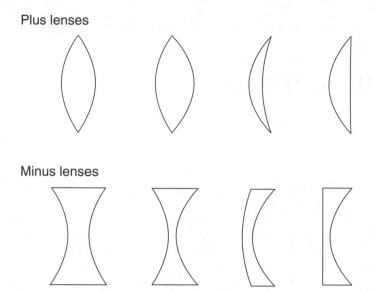

Minus lenses

FIGURE 4-1. Common shapes of lenses. The plus lenses (from left to right) are equiconvex, biconvex, plus meniscus, and planoconvex. The minus lenses (from left to right) are equiconcave, biconcave, minus meniscus, and planoconcave.

light rays travel from left to right, the secondary focal point is (1) the point to which the light rays converge or (2) the point from which they appear to originate (Fig. 4-3A). The primary focal point is located by reversing the direction of light so that the parallel rays travel from right to left (Fig. 4-3B).

The focal lengths are determined with the same relationship that is used for spherical surfaces:

$$P = -n/f = n'/f'$$

Unlike the case with a spherical surface, the index of refraction of the thin lens material (e.g., plastic, glass) is not used to determine the secondary focal length. Rather, this focal length is calculated using the index of the substance to the right of the lens. When the lens is surrounded by a single medium (such as air), $n = n'$. In this case,

$$P = -n/f = n/f'$$

Let us look at an example. *Locate the primary and secondary focal points for a lens that has a power of +3.00 D when it is located in air.* For this lens in air, we have (Fig. 4-4):

$$P = n / f'$$

$$f' = (100)(1.00) / +3.00 \text{ D}$$

$$f' = +33.33 \text{ cm}$$

A

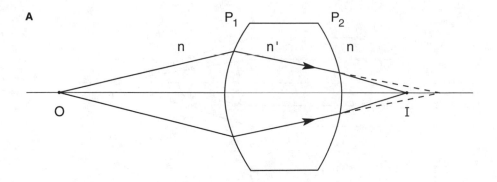

B Plus thin lens

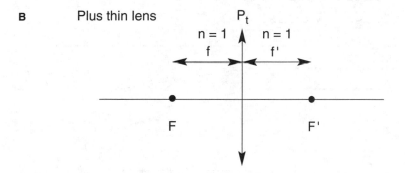

Minus thin lens

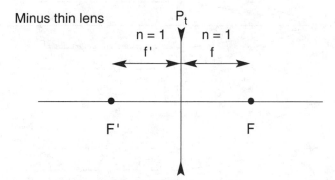

FIGURE 4-2A. A lens is formed by two spherical surfaces. Refraction occurs at each of the two surfaces. If treated as a thin lens, the total power (P_T) is the sum of the powers of the front surface (P_1) and back surface (P_2) of the lens. **B.** Schematic representations of a thin plus lens (top) and a thin minus lens. The front and back surfaces are collapsed to a single plane—a vertical line— where all refraction is assumed to occur. The power of the thin lens (P_T) is the sum of the powers of its front and back surfaces.

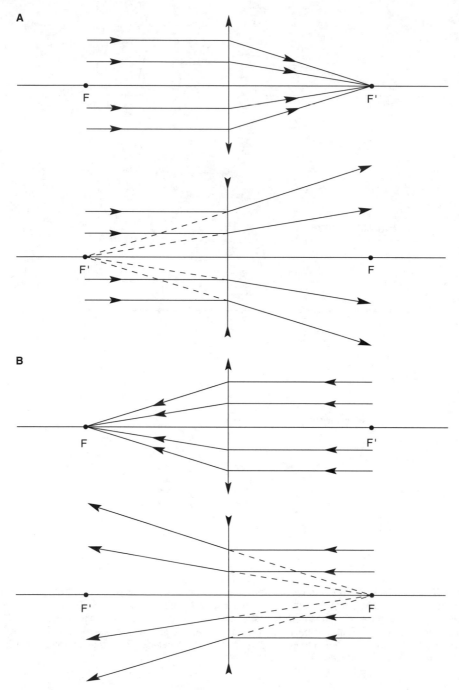

FIGURE 4-3A. Determination of the secondary focal points for a plus (top) and a minus lens. **B.** Determination of the primary focal points for a plus and a minus lens.

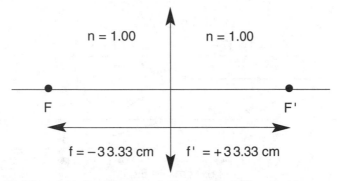

FIGURE 4-4. When a thin lens is surrounded by a single medium (in this case, air), $f = f'$.

The secondary focal point for this converging lens is located 33.33 cm to the right of the lens. The absolute values of the secondary and primary focal lengths are equal to each other because the secondary and primary refractive media are the same (i.e., air).

RAY TRACING

The same principles that we learned for ray tracing with spherical surfaces apply to thin lenses. Figure 4-5 shows a real image formed by a plus lens, a virtual image formed by a plus lens, and a virtual image formed by a minus lens. **Note that a plus lens forms a real image when the (real) object is located beyond the focal length and a virtual image when the object is located within the focal length.**[2]

PARAXIAL RELATIONSHIP

As with spherical surfaces, the paraxial relationship is convenient for locating images and determining magnification. Since the primary and secondary media are usually the same, it is generally more straightforward to solve optical problems for thin lenses.

Consider a +10.00 D lens that is used to magnify the printed words on a page located 9.00 cm from the lens. Where is the image located and what is the lateral magnification? First, draw a diagram (Fig. 4–6). The object is located within the focal length of the lens. Although the light rays' divergence is diminished

---

[2] For an object located at the primary focal point of a plus lens, a virtual image is formed at infinity. This is discussed in more detail in Chapter 12.

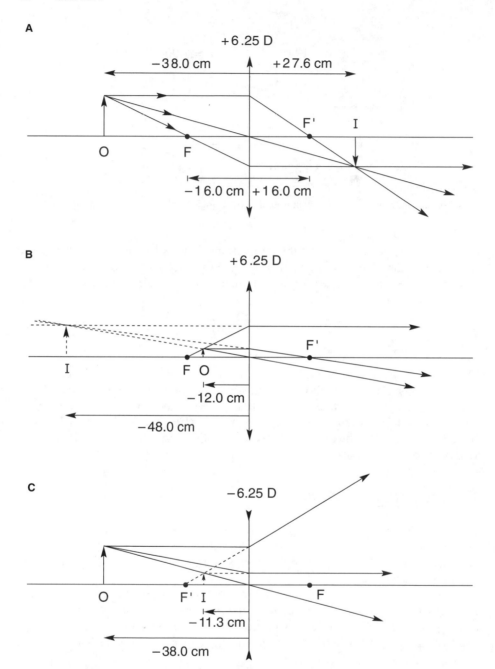

FIGURE 4-5. When drawn to scale, ray tracing can be used to locate images and to determine magnification for a thin lens in much the same manner as for a spherical surface. For a thin lens, the center can be considered to be at the intersection of the lens and the axis. **A.** An object located outside of the primary focal length of a plus lens results in a real, inverted, and minified image. **B.** An object located within the primary focal length of a plus lens results in a virtual, erect, and enlarged image. **C.** The image formed by a minus lens is virtual, erect, and minified.

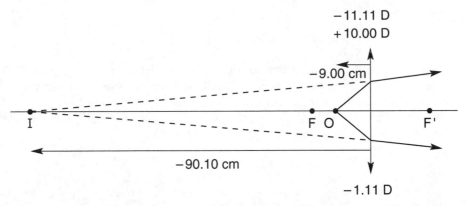

FIGURE 4-6. A plus lens produces a virtual image when the object is located within the primary focal length (*f* = 10.00 cm). The object vergence and lens power are given at the top of the lens, and the image vergence is given at the bottom of the lens.

subsequent to their refraction by the plus lens, they continue to diverge, thereby forming a virtual image. The object vergence is

$$L = n/l$$
$$L = 1.00/l \text{ (where } l \text{ is in meters)}$$

or

$$L = 100/l \text{ (where } l \text{ is in centimeters)}$$
$$L = 100 \ (1.00)/{-9.00} \text{ cm} = -11.11 \text{ D}$$

The paraxial relationship gives us

$$L' = L + P$$
$$L' = -11.11 \text{ D} + 10.00 \text{ D}$$
$$L' = -1.11 \text{ D}$$

The negative image vergence confirms that the image is virtual.[3] Since the lens is surrounded by air (*n* = *n'* = 1.00), the image distance is

$$L' = n \ / \ l'$$
$$l' = (100) \ (1.00)/{-1.11} \text{ D} = -90.10 \text{ cm}$$

The virtual image is located 90.10 cm to the left of the thin lens.

As with a spherical surface, the lateral magnification is given by

$$M_L = L/L'$$

---

[3] An image formed by rays with negative vergence (i.e., diverging rays) is always virtual, and an image formed by rays with positive vergence (converging rays) is always real.

In this example,

$$M_{\rm L} = -11.11 \text{ D}/-1.11 = +10.00X$$

These calculations tell us that an object located 9.00 cm from a +10.00 D lens results in a virtual image that is: (1) 90.01 cm from the lens, (2) on the same side of the lens as the object, and (3) ten times the size of the object.

When a thin lens is located in air (or any other one medium), the formula for lateral magnification can be simplified as follows:

$$M_{\rm L} = L/L'$$

$$M_{\rm L} = \frac{n/l}{n'/l'}$$

Since n is equal to n',

$$\boldsymbol{M_{\rm L} = l'/l}$$

Keep in mind that this relationship is valid only when the medium is the same on both sides of a thin lens.

NEWTON'S RELATION

As we have learned, when a thin lens is located in air (or any other single substance), the primary and secondary focal lengths are equidistant from the lens. This is the basis for *Newton's relation*, which is useful for locating objects and images with respect to the focal points. In Figure 4–7, an object is located at the distance x from the primary focal point of a thin lens and the image is located at a distance x' from the secondary focal point. (The distances x and x' are sometimes refered to as *extrafocal distances*.) From similar triangles, we see that

$$\overline{AB}/\overline{DE} = x/f$$

and

$$\overline{A'B'}/\overline{CD} = x'/f'$$

Since $\overline{AB} = \overline{CD}$ and $\overline{A'B'} = \overline{DE}$,

$$xx' = ff'$$

and since $f = f'$,

$$\boldsymbol{xx' = f^{2}}$$

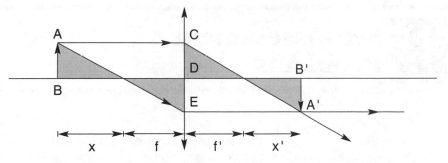

FIGURE 4-7. Relevant distances for Newton's relation. See text for details.

Let us take an example. *An object located 10.00 cm in front of the primary focal point of a lens results in an image that is 40.00 cm to the right of the secondary focal point. What is the power of the lens?* We know that the lens is positive because the image is located to its right. Using Newton's relationship, we find that

$$xx' = f^2$$
$$(10.00 \text{ cm})(40.00 \text{ cm}) = f^2$$
$$f = 20.00 \text{ cm}$$

The secondary focal point of a positive lens is located to its right. Therefore, the lens power is

$$F = 1 / f'$$
$$F = 1 / +0.20 \text{ m}$$
$$F = +5.00 \text{ D}$$

P Self-Assessment Problems

1. A lens made of crown glass has a front surface with a radius of curvature of +8.00 cm and a posterior surface with a radius of curvature of –6.00 cm. (a) Treating this lens as a thin lens, what is its power? (b) Calculate the secondary and primary focal lengths.

2. An object that is 13.00 mm in height is located 15.00 cm from a +20.00 D lens. (a) Using the vergence relationship, locate the image and determine its size. (b) Is the image real or virtual? (c) Is the image erect or inverted?

3. An object that is 30.00 mm in height is located 5.00 cm from a +10.00 D lens. Answer the questions in Problem 2.

4. An object that is 30.00 mm in height is located 10.00 cm from a –30.00 D lens. Answer the questions in Problem 2.

5. A real image is located 50.00 cm from a +25.00 D lens. Locate the object.

6. A virtual image is located 50.00 cm from a +25.00 D lens. Locate the object.

7. A virtual image is located 10.00 cm from a –5.00 D lens. Locate the object.

8. A object that is located 25.00 cm from the anterior focal point of a plus lens forms a real image that is 40.00 cm from the secondary focal point. What is the power of the lens?

Optical Systems with Multiple Surfaces

In the optical systems we have considered up to now, refraction occurs at a single surface (spherical refracting surfaces) or is assumed to occur at a single plane (thin lenses). Most optical systems, however, consist of more than one refracting surface. A series of thin lenses and thick lenses are both examples of optical systems with multiple refracting surfaces (Fig. 5-1).

MULTIPLE THIN LENS SYSTEMS

The simplest multiple-surface optical system is a series of thin lenses that are assumed to have no significant separation between them (Fig. 5-2). The total power of such a system is the sum of the power of the various lenses.

In actuality, of course, there may be a physical gap between two thin lenses; this separation can have a substantial effect on the refractive properties of the lens system. Let us consider an example. *A −5.00 D thin lens is positioned 2.00 cm in front of a +15.00 D thin lens. An object is located 15.00 cm in front of the −5.00 D lens. Locate the image with respect to the +15.00 D lens. If the object is 7.00 cm in height, what is the image's size? Is the image real or virtual? Is it erect or inverted? (Assume that the optical system is in air.)*

With this type of problem, it is more important than ever to draw a diagram (Fig. 5-3). We approach the optical system surface by surface, one surface at a time. The first surface is the −5.00 D thin lens. To locate the image produced by this thin lens, we use the vergence relationship. First, we determine the object vergence:

$$L = n/l$$
$$L = (100)\ (1.00)/-15.00\ \text{cm} = -6.67\ \text{D}$$

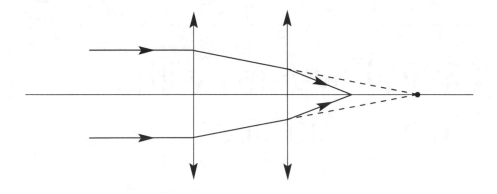

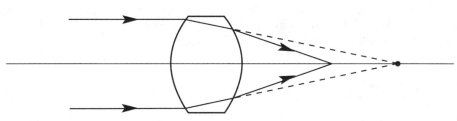

FIGURE 5-1. A series of thin lenses (top) and a thick lens are examples of optical systems with multiple refracting surfaces.

Substituting in the vergence relationship, we have

$$L' = L + P$$
$$L' = -6.67 \text{ D} + (-5.00 \text{ D})$$
$$L' = -11.67 \text{ D}$$

This virtual image is located in front of the first lens. The image distance is

$$L' = n/l'$$
$$l' = n/L'$$
$$l' = (100)\ (1.00)/-11.67 \text{ D} = -8.57 \text{ cm}$$

The image is located 8.57 cm to the left of the first lens. **(In Fig. 5-3, the object vergence and lens power are shown on the top of a lens, and the image vergence is given on the bottom of a lens. We will follow this convention in the remainder of this book.)**

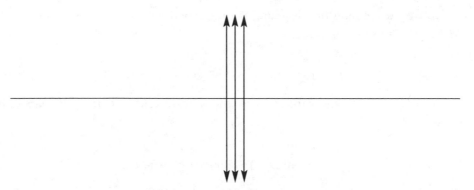

FIGURE 5-2. When there is no significant distance between thin lenses, the total power is the sum of powers of the individual thin lenses.

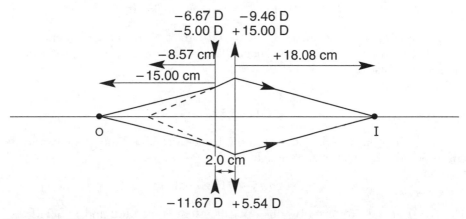

FIGURE 5-3. This optical system, which consists of a thin minus lens followed by a thin plus lens, forms a real image. The object vergence and lens power are given on the top of each thin lens and the image vergence on the bottom of each thin lens.

What is the lateral magnification produced by the first lens?

$$M_L = L/L'$$
$$M_L = -6.67 \text{ D}/-11.67 \text{ D} = +0.57X$$

Therefore, the image size is

$$(7.00 \text{ cm}) (+0.57) = +3.99 \text{ cm}$$

This (erect and minified) virtual image serves as an object for the second lens (i.e., the +15.00 D lens). Light rays diverge from this image, which is located 10.57 cm (8.57 cm + 2.00 cm = 10.57 cm) in front of the second lens. You should confirm this by examining the diagram. At the second lens, these rays produce an *object vergence* of

$$L = n/l$$
$$L = (100) (1.00)/ -10.57 \text{ cm} = -9.46 \text{ D}$$

To locate the image produced by the second lens, we use the paraxial relationship

$$L' = L + P$$
$$L' = -9.46 \text{ D} + (+15.00 \text{ D}) = +5.54 \text{ D}$$

Since the rays that emerge from the lens are converging (they have positive vergence), the image is real. What is its distance from the second lens?

$$L' = n/l'$$
$$l' = (100) (1.00)/+5.53 \text{ D} = +18.08 \text{ cm}$$

The final image is located 18.08 cm to the right of the +15.00 D lens.

What is the size of the final image? The lateral magnification produced by the second lens is

$$M_L = L/L'$$
$$M_L = -9.46 \text{ D}/+5.54 \text{ D} = -1.71X$$

Since the object for this lens (i.e., the image formed by the first lens) is 3.99 cm in height, the final image's height is

$$(3.99 \text{ cm}) (-1.71) = -6.8 \text{ cm}$$

The (real) image produced by this optical system is inverted and minified relative to the initial object.

An alternative approach to determine the final image size is to calculate the lateral magnification for the system as a whole and multiply this total magnification by the initial object size. The lateral magnification for the system is determined by multiplying the magnification of the first surface by the magnification produced by the second surface, thus:

$$\text{Total magnification} = (+0.57) (-1.71) = -0.97X$$

Substituting, we have

$$\text{Final image size} = (+7.00 \text{ cm}) (-0.97) = -6.8 \text{ cm}$$

Consider another example. *An object is located 33.33 cm in front of a +10.00 D thin lens that is located 50.00 cm in front of −2.00 D thin lens. Locate the image, and calculate the magnification.* Viewing Figure 5-4, we see that an object vergence of −3.00 D is incident upon the first lens, resulting in an image

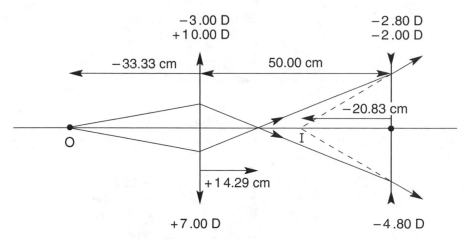

FIGURE 5-4. A virtual image is formed by this optical system.

vergence of +7.00 D. The image is real and is located 14.29 cm to the right of the first lens or 35.71 cm in front of the second lens.

The real image formed by the first lens serves as an object for the second lens. This object emits diverging light rays that are incident upon the second lens with an object vergence of –2.80 D. The image vergence of the rays leaving the second lens is –4.80 D. The image, which is virtual, is located 20.83 cm to the left of the second lens. The final image magnification is

$$\text{Total magnification} = (-3.00D/+7.00D)(-2.80D/-4.80D) = -0.25X$$

The minus sign confirms that the final image is inverted. Note that the image is minified.

VIRTUAL OBJECTS

The best way to understand virtual objects is to solve a problem. *Figure 5-5 shows a two-lens optical system consisting of a +4.00 D thin lens followed by a –2.00 D thin lens. The lenses are separated by 28.00 cm. An object 10.00 cm in height is located 66.67 cm in front of the first lens. Locate the final image, calculate its size, and determine if it is real or virtual and erect or inverted.*

The object vergence at the first thin lens is

$$L = n/l$$
$$L = (100)(1.00)/-66.67 \text{ cm} = -1.50 \text{ D}$$

The image vergence for the first lens is calculated as

$$L' = L + P$$
$$L' = -1.50 \text{ D} + (+4.00 \text{ D}) = +2.50 \text{ D}$$

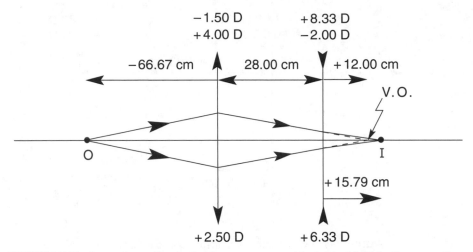

FIGURE 5-5. The image formed by the first lens serves as a virtual object (VO) for the second lens.

Therefore, the image location is

$$L' = n/l'$$
$$l' = (100)\ (1.00)/+2.50\ \text{D} = +40.00\ \text{cm}$$

This real and inverted image *would* be located 40.00 cm to the right of the first lens. The image is not actually formed, however, because the rays that would form it pass through the second lens and are refracted. The image that would have been formed 12.00 cm to the right of the second lens (40.00 cm − 28.00 cm = 12.00 cm) is considered a *virtual object* for the second lens. You can think of a virtual object as the real image that would have been formed by the first lens *if* the second lens did not get in the way. A virtual object has positive vergence and can be formed only by a converging surface or lens.

What is the *object* vergence that is incident on the second lens? Since the rays would have been focused 12.00 cm to the right of the second lens, the object vergence at the second lens is

$$L = n/l$$
$$L = (100)\ (1.00)/+12.00\ \text{cm} = +8.33\ \text{D}$$

The *image* vergence produced by the second lens is

$$L' = L + P$$
$$L' = +8.33\ \text{D} + (-2.00\ \text{D}) = +6.33\ \text{D}$$

Since the vergence is positive, the final image is real and to the right of the second lens. We calculate this distance as

$$L' = n/l'$$

$$l' = (100) \ (1.00)/+6.33 \ D = +15.79 \ cm$$

To determine the size of the final image, we first calculate the total lateral magnification by multiplying the lateral magnification produced by the first lens by the lateral magnification produced by the second lens:

$$\text{Total magnification} = (-1.50D/+2.50 \ D) \ (+8.33 \ D/+6.33 \ D) = -0.79X$$

Therefore the final image height is

$$(10 \ cm) \ (-0.79) = -7.90 \ cm$$

The minus sign tells us that *relative to the original object*, the final image is inverted.

THICK LENSES

The multiple-surface optical systems that we have considered thus far consist of thin lenses. A thick lens, as illustrated in Figure 5-6, also has multiple surfaces: the first and second surfaces of the lens.[1] We can locate the image formed by a thick lens by applying the vergence relationship at each of the surfaces. (In the next chapter, we will learn an alternative approach to solving thick lens problems.)

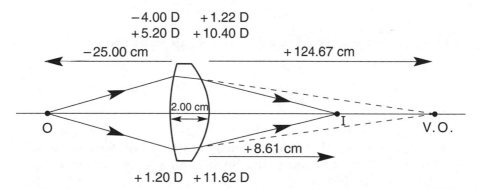

FIGURE 5-6. The image formed by the first surface of this thick lens serves as a virtual object for the second surface. The object vergence and surface power are given on the top of each surface and the image vergence on the bottom of each surface.

---

[1] All lenses have a finite thickness. If a lens is treated as a thin lens, the thickness is ignored. When it is treated as a thick lens, its thickness enters into our calculations. Although treating a lens as a thick lens results in more accurate calculations, it is often acceptable to ignore the lens thickness.

Let us look at a thick lens problem. *An object is located 25.00 cm in front of a biconvex crown glass lens that has an anterior radius of curvature of 10.00 cm and a posterior radius of curvature of 5.00 cm (Fig. 5-6). The lens has a thickness of 20.00 mm. Treating the lens as a thick lens, locate the image with respect to the posterior surface and calculate the magnification produced by the lens. Is the image real or virtual? Is the image erect or inverted?*

The first step is to calculate the powers of the two surfaces. For the anterior surface (e.g., first surface),[2]

$$P = \frac{n' - n}{r}$$

$$P = \frac{1.52 - 1.00}{+0.10 \text{ m}}$$

$$P = +5.20 \text{ D}$$

For the posterior (second) surface,

$$P = \frac{1.00 - 1.52}{-0.05 \text{ m}}$$

$$P = +10.40 \text{ D}$$

The object vergence at the first surface is:

$$L = n/l$$
$$L = (100) (1.00)/{-25.00} \text{ cm}$$
$$L = -4.00 \text{ D}$$

Therefore the image vergence produced by the first surface is

$$L' = L + P$$
$$L' = -4.00 \text{ D} + 5.20 \text{ D}$$
$$L' = + 1.20 \text{ D}$$

The positive vergence tells us that the image is real. Where is the image located? **Since the rays that form the image exist in glass, we use the index of refraction of glass to locate the image.** Using the image vergence, we locate the image as follows:

$$L' = n'/l'$$
$$l' = (100) \, \mathbf{(1.52)}/{+1.20} \text{ D} = +126.67 \text{ cm}$$

---

[2] According to our sign convention, the radius of curvature is positive when the center of curvature is to the right of the surface and negative when it is to the left of the surface.

If the posterior surface did not exist, a real image would be located 126.67 cm to the right of the anterior surface. However, this image is never formed—it serves as a virtual object for the posterior surface (second surface). What is the object vergence at the posterior surface? Taking into account the thickness of the lens, we calculate that the virtual object is located 124.67 cm to the right of the posterior surface (126.67 cm − 2.00 cm = 124.67 cm). **The rays that form this virtual object exist in glass.** Therefore the object vergence at the posterior surface is

$$L = n/l$$
$$L = (100) \, (\mathbf{1.52})/+124.67 \text{ cm}$$
$$L = +1.22 \text{ D}$$

The vergence relationship is used to calculate the image vergence produced by the posterior surface:

$$L' = L + P$$
$$L' = 1.22 \text{ D} + 10.40 \text{ D}$$
$$L' = +11.62 \text{ D}$$

Since the rays are converging, the image is real. Where is it located? **The light rays that form the image live (i.e., exist) in air; therefore we use the index of refraction of air to locate the image:**

$$L' = n/l'$$
$$l' = (100) \, (\mathbf{1.00})/+11.62 \text{ D}$$
$$l' = +8.61 \text{ cm}$$

The final image is located 8.61 cm to the right of the posterior surface.

The total lateral magnification of the thick lens is calculated by multiplying the lateral magnification produced by the first surface by the lateral magnification produced by the second surface:

Total lateral magnification = $(-4.00\text{D}/+1.20 \text{ D})(+1.22\text{D}/+11.62 \text{ D}) = -0.35X$

This calculation confirms that the final image is inverted.

In summary, the light rays that emerge from the object converge after they are refracted by the anterior surface of the thick lens. The posterior surface of the lens converges the light rays even more.

P Self-Assessment Problems

1. A real object, which is 30.00 mm in height, is located 25.00 cm from a crown glass lens that is 30.00 mm thick. The anterior surface of the lens has a radius of curvature of +5.00 cm and the posterior surface has a radius of curvature of −2.50 cm. (a) How far is the image from the back surface of the lens? (b) What is the height of the image? (c) Is the image real or virtual? (d) Is the image erect or inverted?

2. A real object, which is 30.00 mm in height, is located 3.00 cm from a crown glass lens that is 25.00 mm thick. The anterior surface of the lens has a radius of curvature of +12.00 cm and the posterior surface a radius of curvature of −7.00 cm. Answer the questions in Problem 1.

3. A real object, which is 30.00 mm in height, is located 40.00 cm from a crown glass lens that is 30.00 mm thick. The anterior surface of the lens has a radius of curvature of +15.00 cm and the posterior surface has a radius of curvature of +15.00 cm. Answer the questions in Problem 1.

4. Two thin lenses, located in air, are separated by 25.00 mm. The power of the first lens is −10.00 D and the power of the second lens +1.00 D. A real object, which is 45.00 mm in height, is located 30.00 cm in front of the first lens. (a) How far is the image from the second lens? (b) What is the height of the image? (c) Is the image real or virtual? (d) Is the image erect or inverted?

Equivalent Lenses

6

There are two basic approaches that take into account the thickness of a lens. In the previous chapter, a thick lens was considered as a series of independent refracting surfaces. In this chapter, we consider an alternative strategy wherein an optical system with multiple refracting surfaces—such as a thick lens—is replaced by a theoretical lens. This theoretical lens is called an *equivalent lens.*

DEFINITIONS AND FORMULAE

In an equivalent lens, all refraction is assumed to take place at the so-called *principal planes* of the lens.[1] Figure 6-1A shows a thick lens and its (imaginary) principal planes H and H'. Consider light rays that originate from an object, O. The actual path of the rays is given in Figure 6-1B, which shows the refraction that occurs at each of the lens surfaces. Compare this with the equivalent lens construct in Figure 6-1C, which shows all refraction occurring at the principal planes. When an equivalent lens is used to locate an image, we treat it much the same as a thin lens—we do not consider the index of refraction of the lens itself.

Figure 6-2 shows a thick glass lens situated in air. Labeled are the apices of the front (A_1) and back (A_2) surfaces, the primary (H) and secondary (H') principal planes, and the primary (F) and secondary (F') focal points. This thick lens does not have a single focal length—it has several focal lengths. The focal length can be measured from a principal plane, the anterior surface of the lens, or the posterior surface of the lens. When the focal length is measured from the primary equivalent plane to the primary focal point, it is called the *primary equivalent focal length (f_e),* and when it is measured from the secondary equivalent plane to the secondary focal point, it is called the *secondary equivalent focal length (f_e'). The front vertex focal length (f_n)* is measured from the front surface

---

[1] Formally defined, principal planes are imaginary planes of unit magnification where all refraction is assumed to occur. In a thin lens, the principal planes are coincident; all refraction is assumed to occur in this one plane.

A

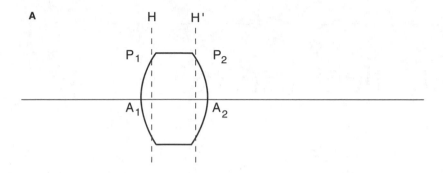

B

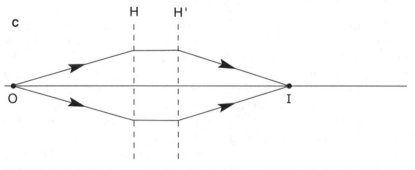

C

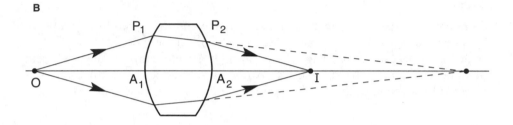

FIGURE 6-1A. A thick lens and its two principal planes. **B.** The actual path of the light rays through the thick lens, showing the refraction that occurs at each surface. **C.** When considered as an equivalent lens, all refraction is assumed to occur at the principal planes.

of the lens to the primary focal point, and *the back vertex focal length* (f_v) is measured from the back surface of the lens to the secondary focal point.

As with a thin lens, the *equivalent power* (P_e) of the thick lens is given by the following relationship:

$$P_e = -n/f_e = n'/f_e'$$

where

$$f_e = \overline{HF}$$

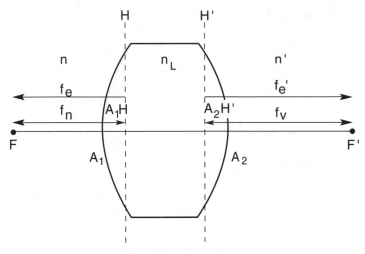

FIGURE 6-2. Various points and distances that are important for understanding thick lenses. See text for further detail.

and

$$f'_e = \overline{H'F'}$$

Again, note that the primary and secondary equivalent focal lengths are specified with respect to the principal planes. When the lens is surrounded by a single medium (i.e., $n = n'$) we have

$$P_e = -n/f_e = n/f_e'$$

Under these conditions, the primary equivalent focal length (f_e) is equal in magnitude to the secondary equivalent focal length (f_e').

Equivalent Power

If we know the powers of the front and back surfaces of a thick lens, we can calculate its equivalent power using a *thick lens formula*. This formula, which takes into account the effect that the lens thickness has on refractive power, is

$$P_e = P_1 + P_2 - cP_1P_2$$

where

$$P_1 = \text{the power of the front surface}$$
$$P_2 = \text{the power of the back surface}$$

and

$$c = t/n_{\mathrm{L}}$$

where

t = the lens thickness in meters
n_{L} = the index of refraction of the lens

Front Vertex and Back Vertex Power

The power of a thick lens can also be specified with respect to its surfaces rather its principal planes (as is the case for the equivalent power). To determine the power of the lens with respect to its front surface—the so-called *front vertex power*, also called the *neutralizing power* (P_{n})—we use the *front vertex focal length*[2]:

$$\boldsymbol{P}_{\mathbf{n}} = -\boldsymbol{n}/\boldsymbol{f}_{\mathbf{n}}$$

where

$$f_{\mathrm{n}} = \overline{A_1 F}$$

The following formula can also be used to determine the *front vertex power.*

$$\boldsymbol{P}_{\mathbf{n}} = \frac{\boldsymbol{P}_2}{1 - c\boldsymbol{P}_2} + \boldsymbol{P}_1$$

To determine the power of the lens with respect to its back surface—the so-called *back vertex power* (P_{v})—we use the *back vertex focal length*:

$$P_{\mathrm{v}} = n'/f_{\mathrm{v}}$$

$$f_{\mathrm{v}} = \overline{A_2 F'}$$

If the lens is surrounded by a single medium (such as air),

$$n = n'$$

and

$$\boldsymbol{P}_{\mathbf{v}} = \boldsymbol{n}/\boldsymbol{f}_{\mathbf{v}}$$

The following formula can also be used to calculate the back vertex power:

---

[2] In determining the front vertex power, light is assumed to travel from right to left (rather than from left to right). Therefore, as we have done before, we insert a minus sign into the formula used to calculate the front vertex power from the front vertex focal length.

$$P_v = \frac{P_1}{1 - cP_1} + P_2$$

The power of the distance prescription of a spectacle lens, as determined with a lensometer, is the *back vertex power*. An ophthalmic lens that is labeled, say, −2.50 DS has a back vertex power of −2.50 DS. Rigid-contact-lens and certain bifocal additions, however, are often specified by giving their front vertex power.

Principal Planes

When the lens is surrounded by a single medium, such as air, the locations of the principal planes (with respect to the lens apices) can be determined with the following formulae:

$$\overline{A_1H} = \frac{ncP_2}{P_e}$$

and

$$\overline{A_2H'} = \frac{-ncP_1}{P_e}$$

where all distances are in meters *and measured from the lens apex* (Fig. 6-2).

The above formulae reveal that the locations of the principal planes depend on the powers of the anterior and posterior surfaces; the shape of the lens determines their locations. Figure 6-3 shows the locations of the principal planes of plus and minus lenses of various shapes.

SAMPLE PROBLEM

Let us return to the example of the thick lens discussed in the previous chapter. *For this thick lens, locate the focal points and principal planes and calculate the equivalent, neutralizing, and back vertex powers*. The lens is redrawn in Figure 6-4. It is biconvex, with a front surface power (P_1) of +5.20 D and a back surface power (P_2) of +10.40 D. It is 20.00 mm thick and made of crown glass. First, we determine its equivalent power:

$$P_e = P_1 + P_2 - cP_1P_2$$

$$P_e = 5.20 \text{ D} + 10.40 \text{ D} - (0.020 \text{ m}/1.52)(5.20 \text{ D})(10.40 \text{ D})$$

$$P_e = +14.89 \text{ D}$$

Plus lenses

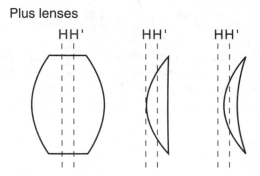

Minus lenses

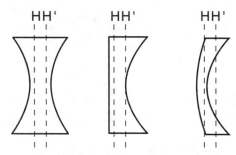

FIGURE 6-3. The positions of the principal planes are dependent on the curvature of the front surface of the lens relative to the curvature of the back surface.

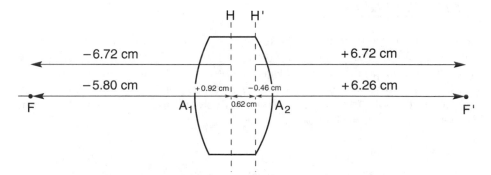

FIGURE 6-4. Various points and distances for the biconvex lens discussed in the text.

The secondary focal point for this converging lens is located to the right of the secondary principal plane. Its distance from the secondary principal plane is

$$P_e = n/f_e'$$

$$f_e' = (100)\ (1.00)/+14.89\ D = +6.72\ cm$$

Since the lens is surrounded by air, the primary equivalent focal length is equal to the secondary equivalent focal length. These focal lengths are measured with respect to the principal planes. We locate the primary principal plane as follows:

$$\overline{A_1H} = \frac{ncP_2}{P_e}$$

$$\overline{A_1H} = \frac{(1.00)\ (0.02\ m/1.52)\ (10.4\ D)}{14.89\ D}\ (1000\ mm/m)$$

$$\overline{AH_1} = +9.2\ mm$$

The primary principal plane is located 9.2 mm to the right of the front lens surface. This is indicated in Figure 6-4. This figure also shows the primary focal length of -6.72 cm (i.e., the distance from H to F).

Now let us locate the secondary principal plane:

$$\overline{A_2H'} = \frac{-ncP_1}{P_e}$$

$$\overline{A_2H'} = \frac{(-1.00)\ (0.02/1.52\ D)\ (+5.20\ D)}{14.89\ D}\ (1000\ mm/m)$$

$$\overline{A_2H'} = -4.6\ mm$$

The secondary principal plane is located 4.6 mm to the left of the posterior surface of this biconvex lens. This distance is labeled on Figure 6-4. Also labeled is the secondary focal length of $+6.72$ cm (the distance from H' to F').

Next, let us determine the neutralizing power. From Figure 6-4, we see that the front vertex focal length is -5.80 cm (i.e., 6.72 cm $-$ 0.92 cm $=$ 5.80 cm). Therefore, the neutralizing power is

$$P_n = -n/f_n$$

$$P_n = -100/-5.80\ cm$$

$$= +17.24\ D$$

Or we can calculate the neutralizing power as follows:

$$P_n = \frac{P_2}{1 - cP_2} + P_1$$

$$P_n = 10.40 \text{ D}/[1 - (0.02 \text{ m}/1.52)(10.40 \text{ D})] + 5.20 \text{ D}$$

$$P_n = +17.25 \text{ D}$$

These same two approaches can be used to calculate the back vertex power. In Figure 6-4, we see that the back vertex focal length is +6.26 cm (i.e., 6.72 cm − 0.46 cm = 6.26 cm). Therefore the back vertex power is

$$P_v = n/f_v$$

$$P_v = 100/+6.26 \text{ cm}$$

$$P_v = +15.97 \text{ D}$$

Or we can calculate the back vertex power as follows:

$$P_v = \frac{P_1}{1 - cP_1} + P_2$$

$$P_v = +5.20 \text{ D}/[1 - (.02 \text{ m}/1.52)(+5.20 \text{ D})] + 10.40 \text{ D}$$

$$P_v = +15.98 \text{ D}$$

We can also calculate the back vertex focal length by treating the thick lens as two independent refracting surfaces (Fig. 6-5). First, we must locate F'. We do this by determining where parallel light rays (originating from an object located at infinity) are focused. For the anterior surface, the object vergence is zero and the image vergence is +5.20 D. Since these rays are refracted in glass, the image distance is

$$L' = n_L/l'$$

$$l' = (100)(1.52)/+5.20 \text{ D}$$

$$l' = +29.23 \text{ cm}$$

The rays converge toward a point that is 27.23 cm (29.23 cm − 2.00 cm = 27.23 cm) to the right of the second surface, forming a virtual object for this surface. These rays live in glass, producing an object vergence at the second surface of

$$L = n_L/l$$

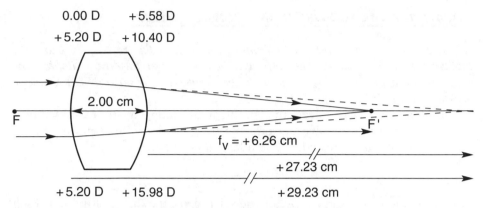

FIGURE 6-5. The secondary focal point of a thick lens can be located by treating the surfaces of the thick lens as two independent refracting surfaces.

$$L = (100)(1.52)/+27.23 \text{ cm}$$

$$L = +5.58 \text{ D}$$

This object vergence (+5.58 D) is incident upon the back lens surface, whose power is +10.40D; therefore the image vergence is +15.98 D. The image rays exist in air. The image location is

$$L' = n/l'$$

$$l' = (100)(1.00)/+15.98 \text{ D}$$

$$l' = +6.26 \text{ cm}$$

An object that is infinitely far from the first surface of the thick lens is focused at a point 6.26 cm to the right of its second surface. This image point is by definition the secondary focal point (*F'*) of the lens. As we have learned, the distance from the back lens surface to the secondary focal point is the back vertex focal length. Note that this surface-by-surface approach gives us the same back vertex focal length as the thick lens approach.[3]

---

[3] The same logic can be used to calculate f_n. Parallel light rays traveling from *right* to *left* are first refracted by the back surface of the lens and then by the front surface; they are focused at the primary focal point. The distance from the front surface of the lens to the primary focal point is the front vertex focal length. The reader should do the
calculations to make sure that he or she understands the important concepts that are necessary to locate this focal point.

LOCATING AN IMAGE USING AN EQUIVALENT LENS

An object is located 25.00 cm in front of the lens in Figure 6-4 (redrawn in Fig. 6-6). Locate the image with respect to the posterior surface and calculate the magnification produced by the lens. Is the image real or virtual? Is the image erect or inverted?

In Chapter 5, we solved this problem by taking a surface-by-surface approach. We can also solve the problem by constructing an equivalent lens. The equivalent lens is treated as a thin lens in air, where

$$n = n' = 1.00$$

In locating the image formed by an equivalent lens, the index of the lens itself is not considered.

Looking at Figure 6-6, we see that the real object is located 25.92 cm in front of the primary principal plane (25.00 cm + 0.92 cm = 25.92 cm). The object vergence at the primary principal plane is

$$L = n/l$$

$$L = (100)(1.00)/-25.92 \text{ cm}$$

$$L = -3.86 \text{ D}$$

Applying the vergence equation, we have

$$L' = L + P_e$$

$$L' = -3.86 \text{ D} + 14.89 \text{ D}$$

$$L' = +11.03 \text{ D}$$

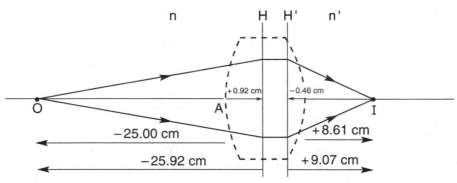

FIGURE 6-6. An image can be located by treating the thick lens as an equivalent lens. All refraction is assumed to occur at the principal planes.

As with a thin lens in air, the image rays exist in air. Therefore the location of the real image with respect to the secondary equivalent plane is

$$L' = n'/l'$$

$$l' = (100)(1.00)/+11.03 \text{ D}$$

$$l' = +9.07 \text{ cm}$$

This real image is located 9.07 cm to the right of the secondary principal plane or 8.61 cm (9.07 cm − 0.46 cm = 8.61 cm) to the right of the posterior surface of the lens. This answer is about the same as the one we obtained with a surface-by-surface approach in Chapter 5.

The equivalent lens approach can also be used to calculate the lateral magnification produced by the thick lens. The formula is the same as that for a thin lens:

$$M_L = L/L'$$

$$M_L = -3.86 \text{ D}/11.03 \text{ D}$$

$$M_L = -0.35X$$

This is the same magnification that we obtained when treating the lens surfaces independently (as we did in Chap. 5). Note that the magnification is negative, confirming that the real image is inverted.

NODAL POINTS

By definition, when a light ray is directed toward the *anterior nodal point, N,* it emerges from the *secondary nodal point, N',* at the same angle with respect to the optical axis (Fig. 6-7). That is, a ray headed toward *N* leaves *N'* with its direction unchanged.[4]

For a spherical optical surface, there is a single nodal point that is located at the surface's center of curvature. A ray directed toward the center of curvature has an angle of incidence of zero degrees—it is not deviated (Figs. 2–8 and 2-9). A thin lens also has only one nodal point, which is located at its *optical center*—the intersection of the lens and the optical axis.

In thick lenses and other complex optical systems, the nodal points are not coincident with each other. For a thick lens that is surrounded by air (or any other single medium), *N* is coincident with *H* and *N'* is coincident with *H'*. This is the case in Figure 6-7.

---

[4] Formally defined, the nodal points are points of unit angular magnification.

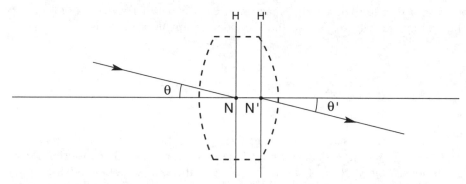

FIGURE 6-7. A light ray headed toward the primary nodal point emerges from the secondary nodal point at the same angle with respect to the optical axis (i.e., $\theta = \theta'$); therefore the direction of the ray is unchanged.

The primary focal point (F), secondary focal point (F'), primary principal point (H), secondary principal point (H'), anterior nodal point (N), and posterior nodal point (N') constitute the *cardinal points* of an equivalent lens.[5] The six cardinal points fully describe the equivalent lens and allow the solution of virtually all optical problems involving paraxial light rays. As we will see in subsequent chapters, the cardinal points can be useful for understanding complex optical systems—such as the eye—that are made up of multiple refracting surfaces.

---

[5] The principal points are located at the intersections of the principal planes and the optical axis.

P Self-Assessment Problems

1. A 30.00 mm-thick biconvex crown glass lens has an index of refraction of 1.52. The front surface has a radius of curvature of +5.00 cm and back surface has a radius of −2.50 cm. The lens is surrounded by air. (a) Calculate P_e, P_v, *and* P_n and determine the following distances: A_1H, A_2H', FH, and $F'H'$. (b) A real object that is 30.00 cm in height is located 25.00 cm in front of the lens. Treating the optical system as an *equivalent lens*, locate the image with respect to A_2 and determine its size. (c) Using a *surface-by-surface approach*, locate the image with respect to A_2 and determine its size.

2. A crown glass lens has a front surface radius of curvature of +25.00 mm and a back surface radius of curvature of +75.00 mm. The lens is 10.00 mm thick and located in air. (a) Calculate P_e, P_v, *and* P_n and calculate the following distances: A_1H, A_2H', FH, and $F'H'$. (b) A real object that is 1.00 cm in height is located 15.00 cm in front of the lens. Treating the optical system as an *equivalent lens*, locate the image with respect to A_2 and determine its size. (c) Using a *surface-by-surface approach*, locate the image with respect to A_2 and determine its size.

Schematic Eyes and Ametropia

7

The eye is a complex optical system consisting of multiple refracting surfaces. To solve certain optical problems, it is necessary to consider the optical properties of the eye in all their complexity. For many optical problems and clinical cases, however, a satisfactory solution can be obtained by using a simplified optical model of the eye. These simplified optical models are referred to as *schematic eyes*.

Gullstrand and Reduced Eye Models

Figure 7-1A illustrates the *Gullstrand # 1 eye,* also referred to as the **exact eye.** This model eye has six refracting surfaces: the anterior and posterior surfaces of the cornea (*n* = 1.376), lens cortex (*n* = 1.387), and lens nucleus (*n* = 1.406).[1] The *Gullstrand # 2 eye (simplified eye),* illustrated in Figure 7-1B, is a further simplification. This model eye has only three surfaces: a single corneal surface and two crystalline lens surfaces.

For most day-to-day clinical applications, it not necessary to use the Gullstrand #1 or #2 eyes. Rather, we use the so-called *reduced eye* (Fig. 7-1C), for which all refraction is assumed to occur at a single surface.[2] This surface separates air from the aqueous (*n* = 1.333) and is located 1.67 mm to the right of the corneal surfaces of the exact and simplified eyes. There is a single nodal point located at the center of curvature of the refracting surface (radius = 5.55 mm).

---

[1] The index of refraction of the crystalline lens is not uniform: it varies continuously from the lens surface to it core.

[2] This surface is coincident with the two principal planes. These two planes are coincident with each other, as is the case for all single-surface refracting systems and thin lenses.

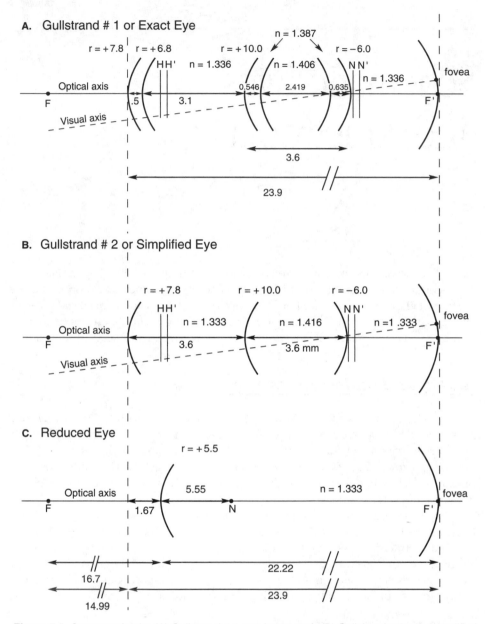

Figure 7-1. Constants for the (A) Gullstrand # 1 eye (exact eye), (B) Gullstrand # 2 eye (simplified eye), and (C) reduced eye. All distances are in millimeters.

Emmetropia

A real object is located infinitely far from the surface of the reduced eye.[3] Where is the image located?

First, let us calculate the power of the refracting surface of the reduced eye (Fig. 7-1C):

$$P = \frac{n' - n}{r}$$

$$P = \frac{1.333 - 1.00}{0.00555 \text{ m}}$$

$$P = +60.00 \text{ D}$$

The object, which is located at infinity, has zero vergence. Following refraction by the surface of the reduced eye, the image vergence is

$$L' = L + P$$
$$L' = 0 + 60.00 \text{ D}$$
$$L' = +60.00 \text{ D}$$

Since the image rays exist in aqueous, the image distance is calculated as

$$L' = n'/l'$$
$$l' = (1.00)(1.333)/+60.00 \text{ D}$$
$$l' = +0.0222 \text{ m}$$
$$l' = +22.22 \text{ mm}$$

The infinitely distant object is focused 22.22 mm from the refracting surface (Fig. 7-2). From Figure 7-1C, we know that the axial length of the reduced eye is

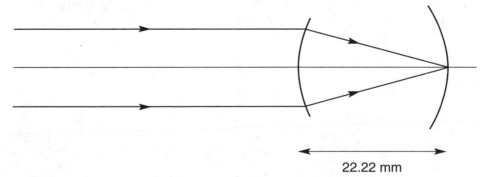

22.22 mm

Figure 7-2. In the emmetropic reduced eye, an infinitely distant object is imaged on the retina.

---

[3] The refractive surface of the reduced eye is located 1.67 mm to the right of the cornea. We will ignore this small distance and assume that the refractive surface of the reduced eye is coincident with the cornea.

22.22 mm; therefore the image is focused on the retina. This is the definition of *emmetropia*. Defined more formally, in the emmetropic eye the retina is conjugate with infinity.

Myopia

Consider an eye that is too long—it has an axial length length of 23.22 mm rather than 22.22 mm. The eye's power is +60.00 D. We know that an infinitely distant object is focused 22.22 mm behind the refracting surface, or 1.00 mm anterior to the retina of this eye. **By definition, the eye is *myopic*: an infinitely distant object is focused anterior to the retina** (Fig. 7-3A).[4]

Where must an object be located if its image is to be focused on the retina of a reduced eye that has an axial length of 23.22 mm and power is +60.00 D? (In this and the other examples in this chapter, we assume that the accommodation of the eye is fully relaxed and the accommodative power is zero. Accommodation is discussed in the next chapter.)

Refer to Figure 7-3B. If the image is focused on the retina, the image vergence must be[5]

$$L' = n'/l'$$
$$L' = (1000)(1.333)/+23.22 \text{ mm}$$
$$L' = +57.41 \text{ D}$$

We use the paraxial relationship to determine the object vergence:

$$L' = L + P$$
$$+57.41 \text{ D} = L + 60.00 \text{ D}$$
$$L = -2.59 \text{ D}$$

Light rays with a vergence of −2.59 D are focused on the retina. **This is referred to as the *far-point vergence*, and the eye is said to be 2.59 D myopic**. To produce this vergence, the object must be located in front of the cornea. The distance from the cornea to the object is[6]

$$L = n/l$$
$$l = (100)(1.00)/- 2.59 \text{ D}$$
$$l = -38.61 \text{ cm}$$

An object that is located 38.61 cm in front of the cornea is focused on the retina. This point is defined as the *far point of the eye* (FP), and, in a myopic eye, is located anterior to the cornea. The far point is conjugate with the retina.

---

[4] A patient who is myopic has the condition of *myopia*.

[5] We have placed a factor of 1000 in the numerator because we are keeping the axial length in millimeters.

[6] Because we have placed a factor of 100 in the numerator, the calculated distance is in centimeters.

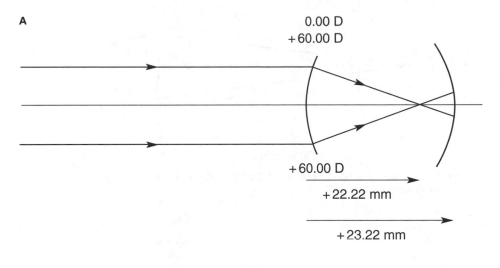

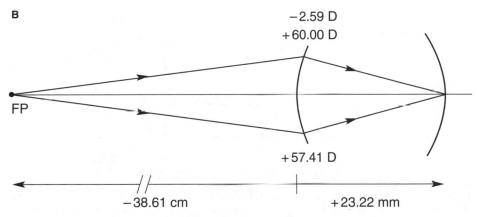

Figure 7-3A. In myopia, an infinitely distant object is imaged anterior to the retina. **B.** An object that is located at the far point of the eye is imaged on the retina. The far point is conjugate with the retina.

Objects located further from the cornea than the far point are focused anterior to the retina (Fig. 7-4).

What power corrective lens is required to image an infinitely distant object on the retina of this myopic eye? If the lens is placed in the plane of the cornea, its power must be –2.59 D. When light rays from an infinitely distant object strike this lens, an image is formed at the far point of the eye; this image serves as an object for the eye and is focused on the retina (Fig. 7-5).

A lens corrects myopia by focusing an infinitely distant object at the far point of the eye. The secondary focal point of the correcting lens must be coincident with the far point of the eye.

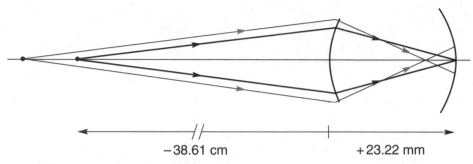

−38.61 cm   +23.22 mm

Figure 7-4. An object that is located further from the myopic eye than the far point will be imaged in front of the retina.

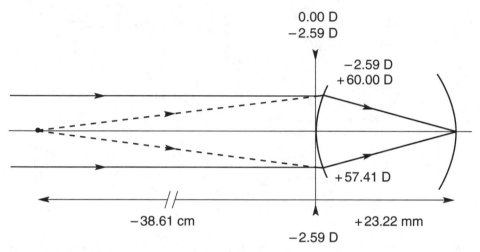

Figure 7-5. A corrective lens images an infinitely distant object at the far point of the eye. Since the far point is conjugate with the retina, a focused image is formed on the retina. Vergence values and dioptric powers are given for both the corrective lens and the eye.

In the myope discussed above, the power of the eye is normal (+60.00 D), but the eye is too long. This is referred to as *axial myopia*. In other cases of myopia, the axial length is normal (22.22 mm), but the eye's refractive power is too strong—a condition labeled *refractive myopia*.

Hyperopia

Just as an eye can be too long, it can also be too short (Fig. 7-6). Consider an eye with an axial length of 21.22 mm and a power of +60.00 D. An object at infinity is focused 22.22 mm behind the cornea, 1.00 mm posterior to the retina

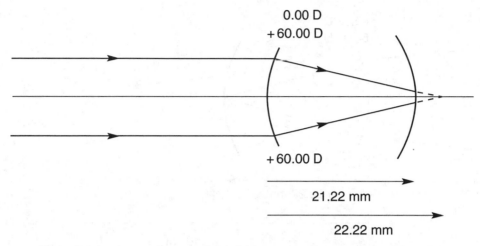

Figure 7-6. In a hyperopic eye, an infinitely distant object is imaged behind the retina.

of this eye. **By definition, the eye is hyperopic: an infinitely distant object is focused behind the retina.**[7]

Where must an object be located if it is to be focused on the retina of a reduced eye with an axial length of 21.22 mm and a refractive power of +60.00 D? If the image is focused on the retina, the image vergence must be

$$L' = n'/l'$$
$$L' = (1000)(1.333)/+21.22 \text{ mm}$$
$$L' = +62.82 \text{ D}$$

To determine the object vergence, we use the vergence relationship

$$L' = L + P$$
$$+62.82 \ D = L + 60.00 \ D$$
$$L = +2.82 \ D$$

Light rays with +2.82 D of vergence are focused on the retina. **This is referred to as the far-point vergence, and the eye is said to be 2.82 D hyperopic.**

Note that the far-point vergence is positive. What does this mean? It means that the object must be located behind the cornea—it is a virtual object (Fig. 7-7A). The light rays that form this virtual object exist in air. The distance from the cornea to the virtual object is

$$L = n/l$$
$$l = (100)(1.00)/+2.82 \text{ D}$$
$$l = +35.46 \text{ cm}$$

---

[7] A patient who is hyperopic has the condition of *hyperopia* (sometimes called *hypermetropia*).

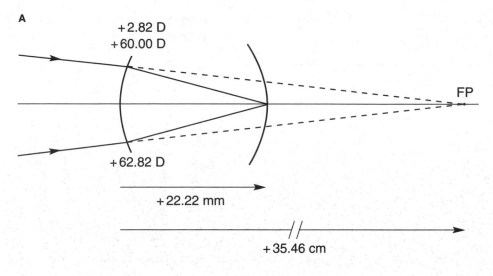

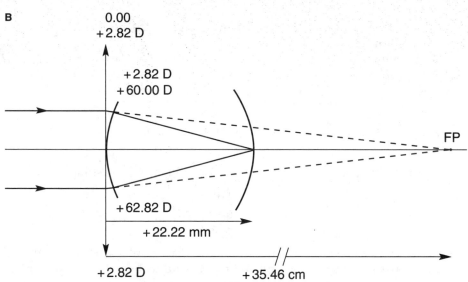

Figure 7-7A. A virtual object that is located at the far point of the hyperopic eye is imaged on the retina. The far point is conjugate with the retina. **B.** A corrective lens images an infinitely distant object at the far point of the eye. Since the far point is conjugate with the retina, a focused image is formed on the retina.

Light rays that are headed toward a point 35.46 cm behind the cornea are focused on the retina. This is the *far point of the hyperopic eye FP*, which is always located posterior to the cornea. The far point is conjugate with the retina.

What power corrective lens is required to image an infinitely distant object on the retina of this hyperopic eye? The lens must form an image at the far point of the eye; this image serves as an object for the eye and is focused on the retina. **Therefore its secondary focal point must be coincident with the far point** (Fig. 7-7B). To achieve this, the lens—when at the plane of the cornea—must have a power of +2.82 D.

With the corrective lens in place, an infinitely distant object is focused on the retina. Without the lens in place, the image will be defocused unless the patient can accommodate +2.82 D. (Accommodation, the process whereby the positive power of the crystalline lens increases beyond its resting power, is discussed in the next chapter.)

In the example that we just discussed, the power of the eye is normal (+60.00 D), but the eye is too short. This is referred to as *axial hyperopia*. In other cases of hyperopia, the length of the eye is normal (22.22 mm), but the refractive power is too weak, a condition labeled *refractive hyperopia*.

Far-Point in Emmetropia

Where must an object be located for it to be focused on the retina of an emmetropic eye (assuming no accommodation)? Since the object must be located at infinity, the far point of the emmetropic eye is at infinity.

Far-Point Vergence Relationship

As we have learned in this chapter, for an object to be focused on the retina of the uncorrected eye, it must produce a vergence that is equal to the far-point vergence. The combination of the far-point vergence and the refractive power of the eye results in an image that is focused on the retina. This condition can be expressed by the following relationship, which we call the *far-point vergence relationship* (Fig. 7-8):

$$A = F_{fp} + P_{eye}$$

Where

$A = 1.333 \, / \, a$, where a is the axial length of the eye

F_{fp} = the far point vergence

P_{eye} = the power of the reduced eye

Let us look at an example. *An eye with a power of +60.00 D has an axial length of 25.00 mm. What power lens, when placed in the plane of the cornea, corrects the refractive error? Locate the far point of the eye.* We can solve this problem by using the far-point vergence relationship (Fig. 7-9):

$$A = F_{fp} + P_{eye}$$

A

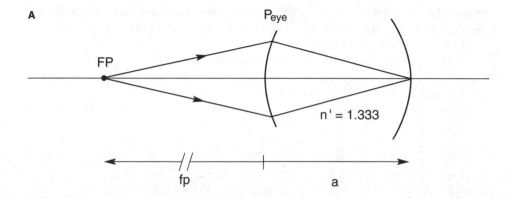

B

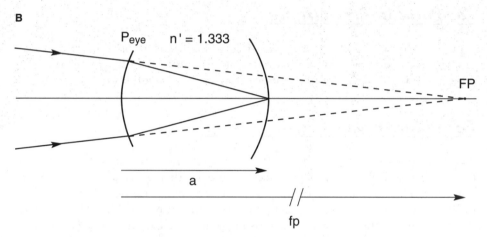

Figure 7-8. The far-point vergence relationship can be used to determine the far-point vergence in (A) myopia and (B) hyperopia. See text for details.

$$1.333/+0.025 \text{ m} = F_{fp} + 60.00 \text{ D}$$
$$F_{fp} = -6.68 \text{ D}$$

By definition, the eye is 6.68 D myopic. For an object to be imaged on the retina, it must have a vergence of –6.68 D at the cornea, which can be produced with a –6.68 D lens in the plane of the cornea.

Where is the far point of this eye?

$$F_{fp} = 1.000 / fp$$
$$-6.68 \text{ D} = 1.000 / fp$$
$$fp = -0.1497 \text{ m}$$
$$fp = -14.97 \text{ cm}$$

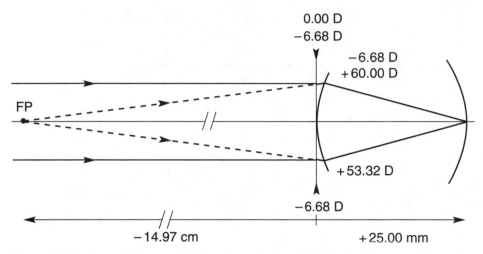

Figure 7-9. The far-point vergence relationship can be used to determine the amount of myopia. See text for details.

An object located 14.97 cm anterior to the cornea of the reduced eye is focused on the retina. Objects located further than 14.97 cm from the eye are out of focus.

Just a slight increase in the axial length can cause clinically significant myopia. *If an eye has 1.00 D of axial myopia, what is its axial length?* We know that the far point vergence is –1.00 D, and the power of the eye is +60.00 D. The far-point vergence relationship gives us the axial length:

$$A = F_{fp} + P_{eye}$$
$$1.333/a = -1.00 \text{ D} + 60.00 \text{ D}$$
$$a = +0.02259 \text{ m}$$
$$a = +22.59 \text{ mm}$$

The axial length is 22.59 mm; it is 0.37 mm too long (i.e., 22.59 mm –22.22 m = 0.37 mm). A rule of thumb is that for every 1/3-mm increase in the eye's axial length, it becomes 1.00 D more myopic. Consequently, an eye that is 1.00 mm too long is approximately 3.00 D myopic.

Myopia and hyperopia are referred to as *refractive errors*. A patient with a refractive error has the condition of *ametropia*.

Lens Effectivity

Let us reconsider the case of a myopic eye that is corrected with a –6.68 D lens placed in the plane of the cornea. Since the lens is in the plane of the cornea,

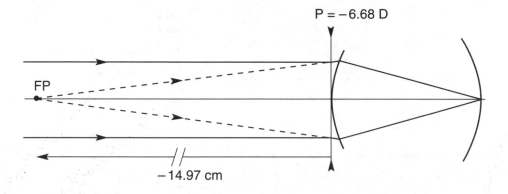

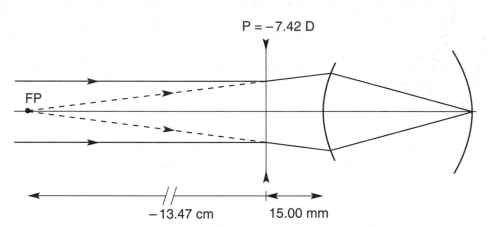

Figure 7-10. This refractive error can be corrected with a −6.68 D contact lens or a −7.42 D spectacle lens.

it must be a contact lens. *We wish to correct the refractive error with a spectacle lens that is located 15.00 mm in front of the eye.[8] What power spectacle lens is required to correct this eye?*

The key to answering this question is to realize that the far point of the myopic eye is a fixed distance from the eye (Fig. 7-10). To correct the refractive error, the secondary focal point of the correcting lens must be coincident with this far point. In the case at hand, the far point is 14.97 cm anterior to the cornea. If the correcting lens is 15.00 mm anterior to the cornea, its secondary focal length must be −13.47 cm (14.97 cm − 1.50 cm = 13.47 cm). The power of a minus lens with a secondary focal length of −13.47 cm is

---

[8] The distance between the cornea and the back surface of the optical correction is called the *vertex distance*.

$$P = 1.00/f$$
$$P = (100)(1.00)/-13.47 \text{ cm}$$
$$P = -7.42 \text{ D}$$

This myope can be corrected with either a –6.68 D contact lens or a –7.42 D spectacle lens at a vertex distance of 15.00 mm. If we replace a myope's contact lens with a spectacle lens, the power must be increased. This only makes sense, since we are moving the corrective lens closer to the far point, thereby requiring the corrective lens to have a shorter focal length.

Consider the case of a myope who notices that distant objects are blurred unless she pushes her spectacles very close to her eyes. How can we explain the patient's symptoms? Most likely, the corrective lenses are not sufficiently strong. By pushing the lenses closer to her eyes, the secondary focal points of the corrective lenses are made coincident with the far points, thereby increasing the lens *effectivity* (Fig. 7-11).

The principles of lens effectivity also apply to hyperopia. *Consider the 2.82 D hyperope who we discussed earlier in the chapter. This hyperope requires a corrective lens of +2.82 D in the plane of the cornea (i.e., a contact lens whose power is +2.82D). What power spectacle lens is required to correct this refractive error? Assume a vertex distance of 15.00 mm.*

The secondary focal point of the corrective lens, whether it is a contact lens or a spectacle lens, must be coincident with the far point of the eye (which is 35.46 cm to the right of the cornea). From Figure 7-12, we see that the secondary focal length of the spectacle lens must be 36.96 cm (35.46 cm + 1.50 cm = 36.96 cm). The power of this spectacle lens is

$$P = 1/f$$
$$P = (100)(1.00)/+36.96 \text{ cm}$$
$$P = +2.71 \text{ D}$$

This hyperope can be corrected with either a +2.82 D contact lens or a +2.71 D spectacle lens. In this example, the difference between the power of the contact lens and the spectacle lens is small. For higher powers, however, lens effectivity is an important clinical factor. For instance, a patient who is corrected with a +10.00 D contact lens requires a spectacle lens whose power is + 8.70 D.

Understanding lens effectivity is critical to understanding common clinical symptoms. *Consider a hyperope who claims that his visual acuity improves when he slides his spectacles down his nose so that they are farther from his eyes. How can we explain this?* Most likely, the lenses—when worn at the normal distance—are not sufficiently strong. By moving the lenses away from his eyes, the hyperope is moving the secondary focal points of the spectacle lenses closer to his far points (Fig. 7-13). (The closer the far point is to the eye, the stronger the lens required to correct the refractive error. In this case, rather than using a stronger lens, the same effect is obtained by moving the lens away from the cornea, thereby increasing its effectivity.)

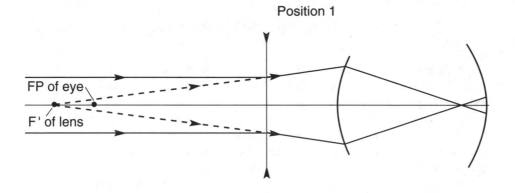

Position 1

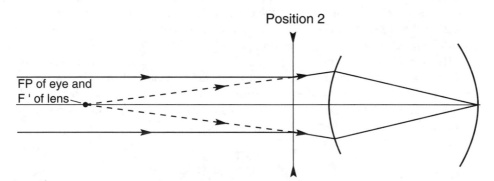

Position 2

Figure 7-11. The effective power of a spectacle lens used to correct myopia is increased by moving the lens toward the eye (from position 1 to position 2).

All of the examples we have discussed up to now involve replacing a contact lens with a spectacle lens. The same principles apply to replacing a spectacle lens with a contact lens. As a practical matter, refractions are almost always performed at the spectacle plane, about 15.00 mm in front of the cornea. Therefore it is more common to calculate the contact lens power from the spectacle power than *vice versa*. You will obtain experience with these calculations when you solve the self-assessment problems at the end the chapter.

CORRECTION OF AMETROPIA WITH LASER AND SURGICAL PROCEDURES

Ametropia is most often corrected with an ophthalmic lens positioned in the spectacle plane or a contact lens in the corneal plane. In recent years, it has

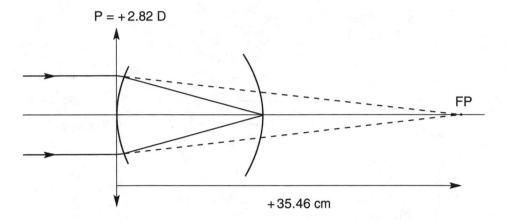

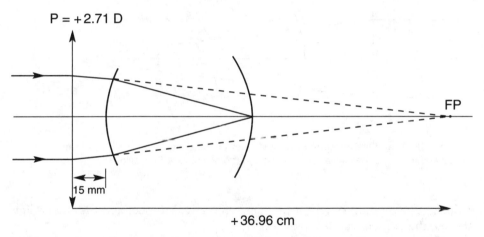

Figure 7-12. This refractive error can be corrected with a +2.82 D contact lens or a +2.71 D spectacle lens.

become commonplace to compensate (or partially compensate) for refractive errors with surgical and laser procedures.

The first widely utilized surgical procedure was *radial keratotomy (RK)*. This procedure is primarily used to compensate for myopia. Radial incisions are made in the cornea, leading to the flattening of this tissue and a resultant decrease in the eye's refractive power (Fig. 7-14).

Photorefractive procedures that utilize excimer laser technology have largely supplanted radial keratotomy. In *photorefractive keratotomy (PRK)*, the corneal epithelium is removed prior to using an eximer laser to sculpt the underlying stroma. In the (currently) more common *laser-assisted in situ keratomileusis (LASIK)*, a microtome is used to create a corneal flap (Fig. 7-15). The exposed stroma is sculpted with the goal of adjusting the refractive power of the eye and

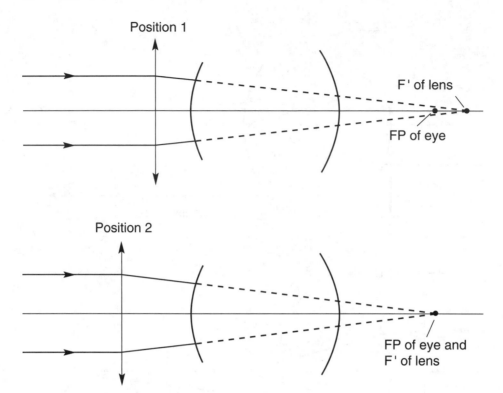

Figure 7-13. The effective power of a plus spectacle lens that is used to correct hyperopia is increased by moving the lens away from the eye (from position 1 to position 2).

reducing the amount of ametropia. Once the laser has sculpted the underlying stroma, the corneal cap is repositioned.

Surgical corneal implants can also be used to compensate for ametropia. The implants can typically be removed if they are unsuccessful in providing an acceptable correction.

In these various laser and surgical procedures, the ametropic correction is in the plane of the cornea. The principles of lens effectivity apply to these laser and surgical corrections in much the same manner as they apply to the correction of ametropia with contact lenses.

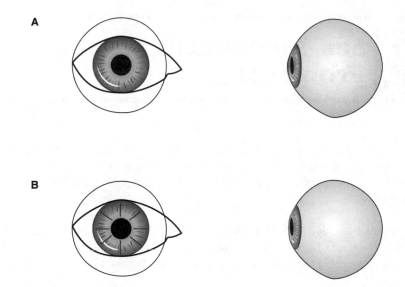

Figure 7-14A. Face-on and profile views of the cornea prior to radial keratotomy. **B.** Following radial keratotomy, the cornea is flattened.

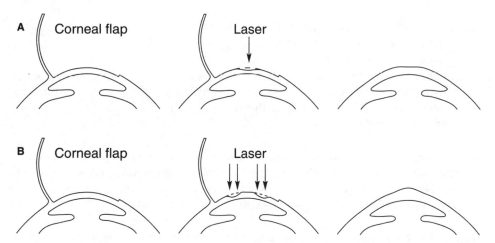

Figure 7-15A. When myopia is corrected with LASIK, the central cornea is flattened. **B.** When hyperopia is corrected with LASIK, the central cornea is steepened.

P Self-Assessment Problems

1. A myopic eye is fully corrected with a –6.00 DS spectacle lens. (a) What is the power of the contact lens required to fully correct this eye? (b) Answer the same question for a hyperopic eye that is fully corrected with a +6.00 DS spectacle lens.

2. A patient's left eye is fully corrected with a –7.00 DS contact lens. (a) What is the power of the spectacle lens required to correct this eye? (b) Answer the same question for an eye that is corrected with a +7.00 DS contact lens.

3. A reduced eye has 10.00 D of myopia as measured at the corneal plane. (a) If the myopia is axial, what is the axial length of the eye? (b) If the myopia is refractive, what is the refractive power of the eye?

4. A reduced eye is corrected with a +5.00 DS spectacle lens. If the ametropia is axial, what is the axial length of the eye?

5. A patient can not see clearly at a distance when viewing with her right eye. The furthest distance at which she can clearly see is 25.00 cm anterior to her cornea (reduced eye). What is the power of the spectacle lens that will correct her ametropia?

6. A patient was last examined 2 years earlier and is currently wearing a –4.00 DS spectacle lens over his right eye. You determine that his far point is 100.00 cm anterior to the spectacle plane. What is the power of the contact lens you would prescribe for this patient to correct his ametropia?

7. An object is located 15.00 cm anterior to the cornea of an emmetropic reduced eye. What is the power of the spectacle lens that is required for the object to be focused on the retina? (Assume the patient cannot accommodate.)

8. An image is located 2.00 mm posterior to the retina of a reduced eye of standard axial length (i.e., 22.22 mm). Where is the object located? (Ignore accommodation.)

Accommodation 8

The eye of an emmetrope (or a fully corrected ametrope) is focused for distance, not for near. The retinal images of near objects will be defocused unless the power of the eye increases. The process whereby the refractive power of the eye increases, thereby allowing near objects to be imaged clearly on the retina, is called *accommodation* (Fig. 8-1). When accommodation is relaxed (i.e., when the eye is focused for distance), the anterior surface of the crystalline lens is comparatively flat and the power of the lens is at a minimum. (Even in this relaxed state, the lens contributes about one-third of the dioptric power of the eye. The cornea contributes two-thirds of the refractive power of the relaxed eye.) During accommodation, the anterior surface of the crystalline lens becomes more curved, thereby increasing the dioptric power of the lens and allowing objects that are close to the eye to be focused on the retina.

The physiology and physical processes of accommodation are complex. The young lens apparently has a natural proclivity to be in a rounded state. When the sphincter-like ciliary muscle is relaxed, the lens zonules are pulled outwards and exert tension at the equator of the lens. This tension causes the anterior surface of the lens to remain flat (Fig. 8-1). When the ciliary muscle constricts during accommodation—much like a sphincter constricting—the tension on the zonules is reduced, thereby allowing the lens to assume its "preferred" rounded shape. In this rounded shape, the curvature of the anterior lens surface is increased and the dioptric power of the eye is increased.

The surface of the lens, referred to as the *lens capsule*, is supple in the young eye. As we age, the lens capsule is thought to become less supple, and this effect may explain the progressive decrease in accommodative capacity that occurs over time. Whereas a 10-year-old child may be able to accommodate 12.00 D (i.e., the total refractive power of the eye increases from +60.00 D for distance to +72.00 D for near), a 75-year-old adult has no ability to accommodate.

When the loss of accommodation leads to clinical symptoms—such as near blur and asthenopia[1]—the condition is referred to as *presbyopia*. Table 8-1 shows

---

[1] *Asthenopia* is another term for eyestrain.

the average maximum accommodative capacity—clinically referred to as the *amplitude of accommodation*—at various ages. Presbyopia is corrected by adding plus lens power to the patient's distance correction. This additional plus lens power is often in the form of a *bifocal add* (see Fig. 11-8).

Presbyopia does not develop at the same rate in all patients. Exposure to high levels of ultraviolet radiation, as occurs with people living close to the equator, appears to accelerate the development of presbyopia.

In the model eyes discussed in the previous chapter, the ciliary muscle is assumed to be relaxed and accommodation is zero. In this chapter, we consider various conditions where accommodation comes into play.

ACCOMMODATION IN THE EMMETROPIC EYE

Accommodation can be represented by a plus lens in the plane of the cornea (Fig. 8-2). The power of this accommodative lens is P_A. **For an object to be focused on the retina, the vergence leaving the accommodative lens must**

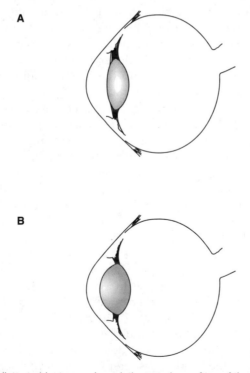

FIGURE 8-1A. When distant objects are viewed, the anterior surface of the crystalline lens is at its flattest, thereby minimizing the lens' refractive power. **B.** When near objects are viewed, the sphincter-like ciliary muscle constricts; this reduces the tension on the zonules, thereby allowing the anterior surface of the lens to bulge forward. As a result, the dioptic power of the lens is increased.

TABLE 8-1. AMPLITUDE OF ACCOMMODATION AS A FUNCTION OF AGE

Age (years)	Typical Amplitude of Accommodation (diopters)[a]
10	12.50
20	9.75
30	7.25
40	4.00
50	2.50
60	1.25
70	0.50
75	0.00

[a]Extrapolated from the data of Donders (1864) and Duane (1912).

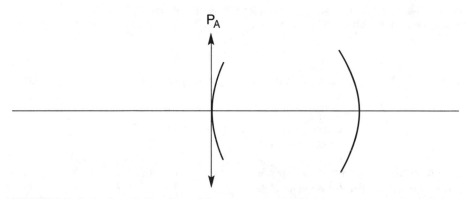

FIGURE 8-2. A plus lens in the plane of the cornea can be used to represent accommodation.

equal the far-point vergence. This can be stated in terms of the *vergence relationship for accommodation*:

$$F_{fp} = L + P_A$$

where

F_{fp} = the far point vergence
L = the *stimulus to accommodation* (i.e., the vergence that the object produces at the cornea)
P_A = the accommodation *as measured in the plane of the cornea* required to focus the object on the retina

Consider an example. *An object is located 33.33 cm in front of the cornea of an emmetropic eye. How much must the eye accommodate to image the object on the retina?* Since the far point of an emmetropic eye is at infinity, the far-point

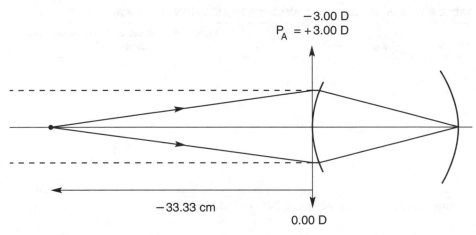

FIGURE 8-3. An object located 33.33 cm anterior to the cornea results in −3.00 D of vergence (at the cornea). For the object to be focused on the retina, the emmetropic eye must accommodate 3.00 D.

vergence is 0.00 D. Substituting in the vergence relationship for accommodation, we have

$$F_{fp} = L + P_A$$
$$0.00\ D = [(100)(1.00)/{-33.33}\ cm] + P_A$$
$$P_A = +3.00\ D$$

The emmetropic eye must accommodate 3.00 D in order for an object at 33.33 cm to be focused on the retina (Fig. 8-3).

This calculation may seem unnecessarily cumbersome. After all, it makes intuitive sense that the emmetropic eye must accommodate 3.00 D to image an object at 33.33 cm on the retina. In subsequent examples, however, we will learn that the determination of the required accommodation is not always so straightforward. To avoid mistakes, it is useful to be methodical in your approach to solving this and all optical problems.

ACCOMMODATION IN UNCORRECTED AMETROPIA

How much must an uncorrected 1.00 D myope accommodate to image the object in the previous example (which is at a distance of 33.33 cm) on the retina?

The object vergence at the plane of the cornea—where accommodation is posited to occur—is −3.00 D. Following accommodation, the vergence must be −1.00 D (Fig. 8-4). From the vergence relationship for accommodation, we have

$$F_{fp} = L + P_A$$
$$-1.00\ D = -3.00\ D + P_A$$
$$P_A = +2.00\ D$$

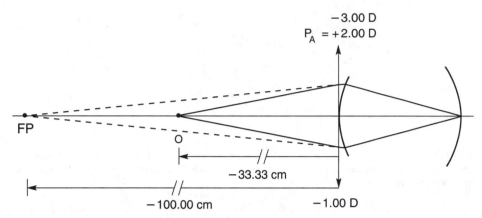

FIGURE 8-4. To image an object located 33.33 cm anterior to the cornea upon the retina, an uncorrected 1.00 D myope must accommodate 2.00 D.

For an object located 33.33 cm anterior to the eye, the uncorrected myope must accommodate less than the emmetrope. This makes intuitive sense because the myopic eye has an excess of plus power—it is too strong for its axial length.[2]

Now let us consider uncorrected hyperopia. *To image the object in the previous example (which is at a distance of 33.33 cm) on the retina, how much must an uncorrected 1.00 D hyperope accommodate?*

Following accommodation, the vergence must be +1.00 D (Fig. 8-6). Using the vergence relationship for accommodation, we have

$$F_{fp} = L + P_A$$
$$+1.00 \text{ D} = -3.00 \text{ D} + P_A$$
$$P_A = +4.00 \text{ D}$$

For an object located 33.33 cm anterior to the eye, the uncorrected hyperope must accommodate more than the emmetrope. This makes sense because the hyperopic eye has less refractive power than the emmetropic eye—it is too weak for its axial length.

Let us summarize the effect of uncorrected refractive error on accommodation. To image a given near object on the retina, the uncorrected hyperopic eye must accommodate the most, the emmetropic eye less, and the myopic eye even less. It is for this reason that the uncorrected myope may continue to have acceptable near vision even as he or she ages and loses the ability to accommodate. For instance, at the age of 65 years, an *uncorrected* 3.00 D myope will still be able to see an object at 33.33 cm clearly, whereas the object will appear

---

[2] How much accommodation is required if an object is located 100 cm anterior to the 1.00 D myopic eye? Since the object is located at the eye's far point, the image is focused on the retina without any accommodation (Fig. 8-5).

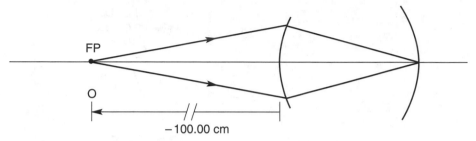

FIGURE 8-5. To image an object located 100.00 cm anterior to the cornea upon the retina, an uncorrected 1.00 D myope does not need to accommodate. The object is located at the eye's far point, which is conjugate with the retina.

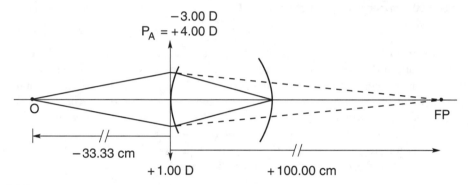

FIGURE 8-6. To image an object located 33.33 cm anterior to the cornea upon the retina, an uncorrected 1.00 D hyperope must accommodate 4.00 D.

blurred to the emmetrope and uncorrected hyperope. (Aging myopes often remove their spectacles to view near objects.)

As he or she ages, the uncorrected hyperope may have difficulty clearly seeing distant objects as well as near objects. *For example, consider the amount of accommodation required for an uncorrected 3.00 D hyperope to image an infinitely distant object on the retina.* For this object to be focused, the patient must either wear a +3.00 D correction or accommodate 3.00 D to compensate for the eye being 3.00 D too weak (Fig. 8-7). A young patient (e.g., 12 years old) will generally be able to accommodate the 3.00 D required to focus distant objects on the retina. Doing so, however, may result in asthenopia (i.e., eyestrain) and/or other symptoms such as intermittent blur. Focusing on near objects will require additional accommodation and may be more difficult and uncomfortable for the patient. As the patient ages and the amplitude of accommodation progressively decreases, the symptoms will become more pronounced. Corrective lenses will alleviate the patient's symptoms.

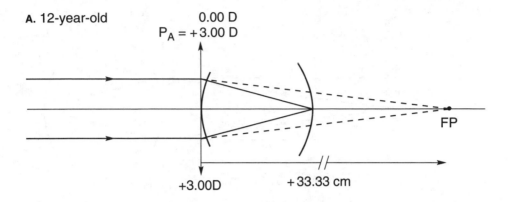

A. 12-year-old

0.00 D
P_A = +3.00 D

+3.00D   +33.33 cm

FP

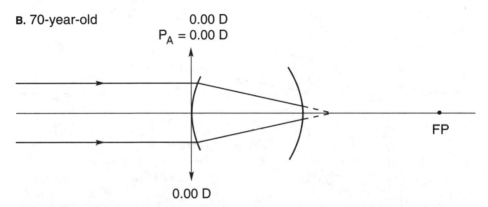

B. 70-year-old

0.00 D
P_A = 0.00 D

0.00 D

FP

FIGURE 8-7A. In viewing a distant object, a 12-year-old uncorrected hyperope can accommodate to focus the image on the retina. The patient may, however, manifest symptoms of asthenopia and/or intermittant blur. **B.** A 70-year-old uncorrected hyperope does not have the ability to accommodate. Therefore the retinal image is out of focus.

NEAR POINT OF ACCOMMODATION

The advantage of myopia for viewing near objects can also be nicely illustrated by determining the closest distance that an object can be from the eye and still be in focus on the retina—the so-called *near point of accommodation* (NPA). *Consider three 50-year-old patients. Each has an amplitude of accommodation of 2.00 D. One patient is an emmetrope, another is an uncorrected 2.00 D myope, and the third is an uncorrected 2.00 D hyperope. Determine the NPA for each patient.*

First consider the emmetrope (Fig. 8-8A). The amplitude of accommodation is 2.00 D and the far-point vergence is zero (i.e., the far point is at infinity). From the vergence relationship for accommodation, we have

A

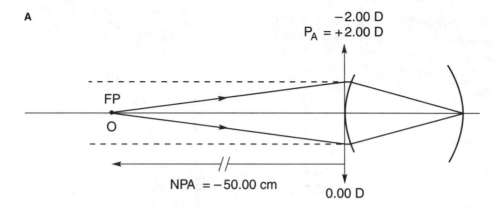

B

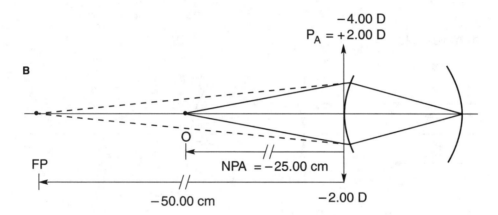

C

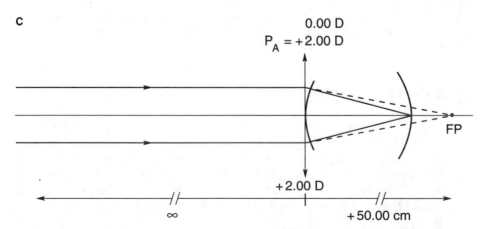

FIGURE 8-8A. The NPA for an emmetrope with an amplitude of accommodation of 2.00 D is 50.00 cm. **B.** The NPA for an uncorrected 2.00 D myope with the same amplitude is 25.00 cm. **C.** The NPA for an uncorrected 2.00 D hyperope with the same amplitude of accommodation is at optical infinity.

$$F_{fp} = L + P_A$$
$$0.00 \ D = L + 2.00 \ D$$
$$L = -2.00 \ D$$

When the eye is maximally accommodated, objects located as close as 50.00 cm ($100/-2.00 \ D = -50.00$ cm) in front of the cornea can be imaged on the retina (i.e., the NPA is 50.00 cm). An object that is closer than 50.00 cm, however, cannot be imaged on the retina because the eye does not have sufficient accommodative power. For instance, for an object located 40.00 cm from this eye to be focused on the retina, the eye would need to accommodate 2.50 D. Since the eye has only 2.00 D of accommodation, the image is blurred.

Now, let us determine the NPA for the uncorrected 2.00 D myope (Fig. 8-8B). The maximum amount of accommodation is the same as it is for the emmetrope (2.00 D), but the far-point vergence is −2.00 D. Therefore,

$$F_{fp} = L + P_A$$
$$-2.00 D = L + 2.00 \ D$$
$$L = -4.00 \ D$$

For this uncorrected myopic eye, the NPA is 25.00 cm: objects located as close as 25.00 cm anterior to the eye can be imaged on the retina. For the emmetrope, an object at 25.00 cm will be out of focus. The uncorrected myopic eye is better able to focus near objects than the emmetropic eye.

Now it's time to look at the 2.00 D uncorrected hyperope who also has an amplitude of accommodation of 2.00 D. Substituting in the vergence relationship for accommodation, we have

$$F_{fp} = L + P_A$$
$$+2.00 \ D = L + 2.00 \ D$$
$$L = 0.00 \ D$$

The NPA is at infinity; consequently, when this hyperope is uncorrected, any object closer than optical infinity will be out of focus (Fig. 8-8C). With the same amplitude of accommodation, an emmetrope has a NPA of 50.00 cm and an uncorrected 2.00 D myope has an NPA of 25.00 cm. The uncorrected myope has an advantage when viewing near objects, whereas the uncorrected hyperope suffers a disadvantage.

ACCOMMODATION IN CORRECTED AMETROPIA

Ametropia can be corrected at the plane of the cornea (with, for example, contact lenses, laser procedures, or orthokeratology) or at the spectacle plane. The amount of accommodation that is required to focus a near object on the retina depends on whether the ametropic correction is in the plane of the cornea or in the spectacle plane.

First consider the case of a myope who is fully corrected with a −5.00 D contact lens. How much accommodation is required to image an object located 10.00 cm anterior to the cornea on the retina? The object vergence at the plane of the cornea is −10.00 D. This object vergence is incident upon the −5.00 D contact lens, resulting in an image vergence of −15.00 D (Fig. 8-9A). For the object

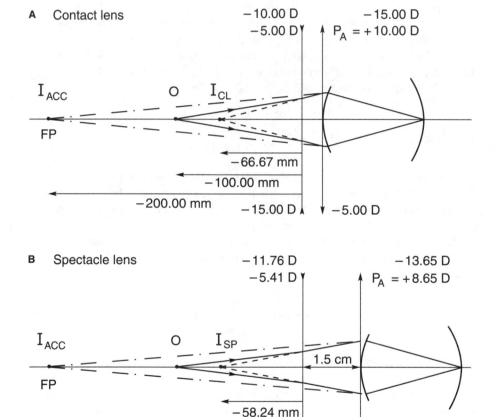

FIGURE 8-9A. To image an object located 10.00 cm anterior to the cornea on the retina, a 5.00 D myope who is fully corrected with a contact lens must accommodate 10.00 D. I_{cI} represents the image formed by the contact lens and I_{Acc} the image formed by the accommodative lens (at the far point). *For illustrative purposes, the figure shows a small gap between the plane of accommodation and the contact lens; this gap does not actually exist.* **B.** To image this object on the retina, the same myope—now corrected with a spectacle lens that is 15.00 mm anterior to the cornea—must accommodate only 8.65D. I_{Sp} represents the image formed by the spectacle lens.

to be focused on the retina, the vergence must be −5.00 D following accommodation (i.e., the far-point vergence). The amount of accommodation required to produce this vergence is given by the vergence relationship for accommodation:

$$F_{fp} = L + P_A$$
$$-5.00 \ D = -15.00 \ D + P_A$$
$$P_A = +10.00 \ D$$

With a correction in the corneal plane, this myope must accommodate 10.00 D—the same amount as an emmetrope—to focus an object that is at a distance of 10.00 cm. *The patient would like to obtain a pair of spectacles to use for those times when she is not wearing her contact lenses.*[3] *What should be the power of the spectacle lenses? When wearing the spectacles, how much accommodation is required to see clearly an object that is located 10.00 cm anterior to the cornea?* In Chapter 7, we learned how to perform calculations involving lens power effectivity. You should confirm that at the spectacle plane of 15.00 mm, the required spectacle lens has a power of −5.41 D.

As shown in Figure 8-9B, the object is located 85.00 mm in front of the −5.41 D spectacle lens. The resulting image vergence is

$$L' = L + P$$
$$L' = [(1.000) \ (1000)/-85.00 \ mm] + (-5.41D)$$
$$L' = -17.17 \ D$$

The vergence leaving the spectacle lens is −17.17 D. Because the lens is 15.00 mm anterior of the cornea, this is not the vergence at the eye. To calculate the vergence at the eye, we must next locate the image formed by the spectacle lens. This image is virtual and located to the left of the spectacle lens. The image distance is calculated as

$$L' = n'/l'$$
$$l' = (1.000)(1.000)/-17.17 \ D$$
$$l' = -58.24 \ mm$$

The virtual image is located 58.24 mm to the left of the spectacle lens and 73.24 mm to the left of the cornea (58.24 mm + 15.00 mm = 73.24 mm). This image is the stimulus to accommodation. Following accommodation, the vergence must be −5.00 D (the far-point vergence). The required accommodation is given by the vergence relationship for accommodation:

$$F_{fp} = L + P_A$$
$$-5.00 \ D = [(1.000) \ (1000)/-73.24 \ mm] + P_A$$
$$P_A = +8.65 \ D$$

---

[3] Patients who wear contact lenses should always have a pair of spectacles as a backup.

When properly corrected with spectacles, this myope must accommodate 8.65 D to see an object located at a distance of 10.00 cm from the cornea. The same myope must accommodate 10.00 D when wearing contact lenses (Table 8-2).[4] This has important clinical implications. Consider a 45-year-old patient who wears spectacles and wishes to be fitted with contact lenses or to undergo a laser procedure. More accommodation is required when the correction is moved to the plane of cornea, and this may lead to asthenopia and/or near blur. It is important for the clinician to be aware that the accommodative demand increases when a spectacle-wearing myopic patient is corrected with contact lenses or a laser refractive procedure.[5]

Now, let us make the same calculations for a hyperope who is fully corrected at distance with a +5.00 D contact lens. When the patient is wearing contact lenses, how much accommodation is required to image an infinitely distant object on the retina? The object is 10.00 cm in front of the +5.00 D contact lens, with a resultant image vergence of −5.00 D (Fig. 8-10A). To produce the far-point vergence (i.e., +5.00 D), the required accommodation is calculated as follows:

$$F_{fp} = L + P_A$$
$$+5.00 \text{ D} = -5.00 \text{ D} + P_A$$
$$P_A = +10.00 \text{ D}$$

When wearing a contact lens, the eye must accommodate 10.00 D—the same amount as an emmetrope.

How much accommodation is required when this hyperope wears her spectacles? Applying the principles of lens effectivity, you should verify that the spectacle lens must have a power of +4.65 D. (The focal length is 200.00 mm + 15.00 mm = 215.00 mm). The object vergence at the spectacle lens plane is −11.76 D,

TABLE 8-2. REQUIRED ACCOMMODATION FOR AN OBJECT LOCATED 10.00 CM FROM THE EYE

Correction in Corneal Plane	Prescription Worn	Accommodation[a]
−5.00 DS	−5.00 DS contact lens	+10.00 D
−5.00 DS	−5.41 DS spectacle lens	+8.65 D
+5.00 DS	+5.00 DS contact lens	+10.00 D
+5.00 DS	+4.65 DS spectacle lens	+11.42 D

[a]As measured in the corneal plane.

[4] You should confirm that when the myopia is *uncorrected*, 5.00 D of accommodation will be required to image the near object on the retina.

[5] To minimize near symptoms, one eye of a bilateral myope is sometimes undercorrected (i.e., the eye remains slightly myopic after it is fitted with a contact lens or following a laser procedure). The undercorrected eye is used to view near objects, and the fellow eye, which is fully corrected, is used to view distant objects. This type of correction is referred to as *monovision*.

resulting in an image vergence of −7.11 D (Fig. 8-10B). The virtual image, which serves as the object for accommodation, is located 140.65 mm to the left of the corrective lens and 155.65 mm to the left of the accommodative plane. To determine the required amount of accommodation, we use the vergence relationship for accommodation, as follows:

$$F_{fp} = L + P_A$$
$$+5.00\ D = [(1.000)(1000)/{-}155.65\ mm] + P_A$$
$$P_A = +11.42\ D$$

Compare these results with those obtained with a myope. Whereas the accommodative demand for a myope decreases in going from contact lenses to

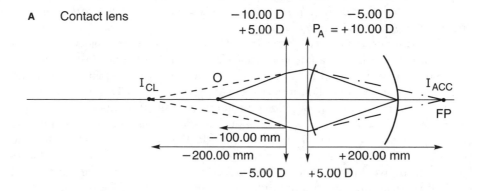

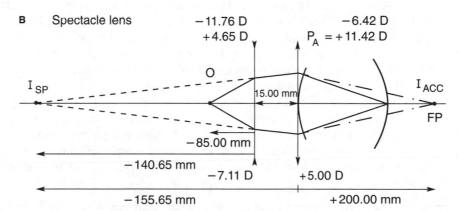

FIGURE 8-10A. To image an object located 10.00 cm anterior to the cornea on the retina, a 5.00 D hyperope who is fully corrected with a contact lens must accommodate 10.00 D. *For illustrative purposes, the figure shows a small gap between the plane of accommodation and the contact lens; this gap does not actually exist.* **B.** To image this object on the retina, the same hyperope—now corrected with a spectacle lens that is 15.00 mm anterior to the cornea—must accommodate 11.42 D.

spectacles, the accommodative demand for a hyperope increases. The results of these calculations are summarized in Table 8-2.

CORRECTION OF PRESBYOPIA

In developed countries, presbyopia probably prompts more visits to the eye doctor than any other single diagnosis. Let us consider an example. *A 48-year-old myope wears −5.00 D spectacles for distance use. When he reads with his distance glasses, he suffers asthenopia and near blur. Although he can take off his glasses to see near objects, it is inconvenient. The patient does most of his near work at a distance of 33.0 cm from the spectacle plane. If the patient has an amplitude of accommodation of 4.00 D as determined at the spectacle plane,[6] what power bifocal add should you prescribe? What is the patient's range of clear vision when looking through the add?*

The patient's *working distance* is 33.0 cm. To image an object located at this distance on the retina, the corrected (for distance) patient must accommodate 3.00 D (as measured in the spectacle—not the corneal—plane). Since the amplitude of accommodation in the spectacle plane is 4.00 D, he is able to do so. The patient, however, cannot comfortably sustain this amount of accommodation because his ciliary muscle is pushed close to its limits. This situation can be improved by prescribing a bifocal add that makes it possible for the patient to use only half his accommodative amplitude when viewing objects located at the working distance. If we prescribe a +1.00 D add, the patient will use half his accommodative amplitude in focusing on objects located at 33.0 cm (i.e., he will accommodate 2.00 D).

When the patient looks through the add with his accommodation totally relaxed, the sum of the add power (+1.00 D) and accommodative power (0.00 D) is +1.00 D. Therefore objects beyond 100.00 cm will be out of focus (Fig. 8-11A). If the patient accommodates fully, the sum of the add power and accommodative power is 5.00 D (in the spectacle plane). This corresponds to a distance of 20.00 cm (Fig. 8-11B). The patient's range of clear vision in looking through the add is from 100.00 to 20.00 cm (as measured from his spectacles).[7]

When the patient uses half his amplitude of accommodation to view a near object, the range of clear vision is *dioptrically* centered on this distance. This is the basis for a clinical procedure often used to determine a patient's add. The doctor selects a tentative add based on the patient's age, and the patient is then instructed to view near-threshold letters located at his near working distance

---

[6] Up to now, we have considered examples where the object distance and NPA are measured with respect to the cornea. In the clinic, these distances are often measured with respect to the spectacle plane. Accommodation is assumed to occur in the spectacle plane—not the corneal plane.

[7] As we will learn in Chapter 11, depth of field increases the range of clear vision.

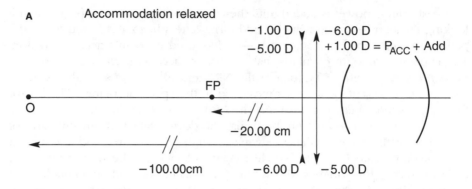

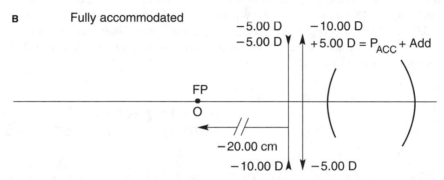

FIGURE 8-11. This fully corrected myope has an amplitude of accommodation, *as measured in the spectacle plane,* of 4.00 D. The patient wears a 1.00 D add. The first lens is the distance correction (a –5.00 D spectacle lens) and the second represents a combination of the add and accommodative powers (i.e., P_{acc} + Add). (Ignore the gap between the lenses—the lenses are separated only for illustrative purposes.) **A.** When accommodation is relaxed (i.e., the accommodative power is zero), the combined add and accommodation have a power of +1.00D. For the object to be imaged on the retina, the vergence leaving the second lens must be equal to the far-point vergence (i.e., –5.00 D); consequently, an object further than 100.00 cm (from the –5.00 DS spectacle lens) will not be focused on the retina. **B.** When the patient fully accommodates, the combined accommodation and add power equal +5.00 D. For the object to be imaged on the retina, the vergence leaving the second lens must be equal to the far-point vergence (i.e., –5.00 D). From the figure, we can see that an object closer than 20.00 cm to the –5.00 DS spectacle lens will not be focused on the retina.

(when looking through the tentative add). The doctor adds plus power to the tentative add until the patient reports that the letters are blurred. This occurs when the patient has fully relaxed his accommodation. The maximum amount of plus that the patient accepts is equal to the amount of accommodation used to resolve the letters through the tentative add and is called *the negative relative accommodation* (NRA).

Next, minus power is added until the letters are blurred. (The patient is still looking through the same tentative add.) The letters become blurred when the patient can no longer accommodate—he has used all of his accommodation. The maximum amount of minus that the patient accepts is *the positive relative accommodation* (PRA). The total of the NRA and PRA is equal to the patient's amplitude of accommodation (as measured in the spectacle plane). The doctor then adjusts the tentative add so that the NRA and PRA are equal.

Let us take an example. Suppose that the doctor selects a tentative add of +1.50 DS for the above patient. Viewing through this tentative add, the patient must accommodate 1.50 D to see clearly letters located at the working distance of 33.0 cm (i.e., the patient's NRA is +1.50 D). When focused on letters located at the working distance, the patient has 2.50 D of accommodation in reserve (i.e., 4.00 D − 1.50 D = 2.50 D); this is the PRA. The goal is to equalize the NRA and PRA. This occurs when the tentative add is changed to +1.00 (making both the NRA and PRA equal to 2.00 D). When viewing letters at the working distance of 33.0 cm through a +1.00 D add, the patient exerts half his amplitude of accommodation, and the range of clear vision is dioptrically centered at the working distance (Fig. 8-12).

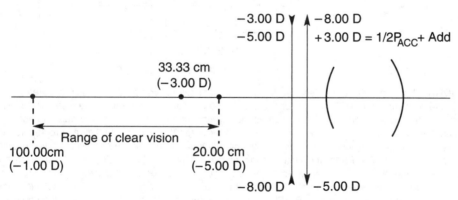

FIGURE 8-12. This presbyopic myope who is fully corrected with spectacles has an amplitude of accommodation of 4.00 D. (This is the same patient as in Fig. 8-11.) Looking through a +1.00 D add, the patient's range of clear vision is *dioptrically* centered on the working distance of 33.33 cm (−3.00 D). The patient can view an object at the working distance and then either relax his accommodation by 2.00 D to clearly see an object 100.00 cm from his eyes or accommodate an additional 2.00 D to see an object 20.00 cm in front of his eyes. (Although the range of clear vision is dioptrically centered on the working distance, it is not linearly centered.)

P Self-Assessment Problems

1. An object is located 10.00 cm anterior to the cornea of a 3.50 D myope (as measured at the corneal plane). How much accommodation is required to image the object on the retina if (a) the patient is uncorrected? (b) corrected with a contact lens? (c) corrected with a spectacle lens?

2. A 5.00 D hyperope (as measured in the corneal plane) views an object that is located 10.00 cm anterior to his cornea. If the patient is wearing a +4.00 DS contact lens, how much accommodation is required to image the object on the retina?

3. An emmetropic presbyope has a range of clear vision from infinity to 20.00 cm from the cornea. What is the power of the contact lens that allows the patient to see clearly at 15.00 cm when using only one-half of her total amplitude of accommodation? (Ignore depth of field.)

4. To image an object located 33.00 cm anterior to his cornea on his retina, an uncorrected 2.00 D hyperope exerts one-half of his accommodative amplitude. What is his amplitude of accommodation? (Ignore depth of field.)

5. An uncorrected 3.00 D myope (as measured at the cornea), views an object that is located 15.00 cm anterior to her cornea through a +1.00 DS lens. If the lens is held 40.00 mm anterior to the cornea, how much accommodation is required to image the object on the retina?

6. A 47-year-old patient is fully corrected in each eye with a –6.00 DS spectacle lens. The patient undergoes LASIK, which fully corrects the ametropia. (a) Prior to the surgery, how much accommodation is required to image an object located 40.00 cm from the cornea on the retina when the patient is wearing his spectacles? (b) Following the surgery, how much accommodation is required to image this same object on the retina? (c) What is the clinical significance of this finding?

Cylindrical Lenses and the Correction of Astigmatism

9

Myopia and hyperopia are spherical refractive errors that, by definition, can be corrected with spherical lenses. The refractive power is the same in each meridian of a spherical lens (Fig. 9-1A). Whether it is measured across the horizontal meridian, the vertical meridian, or anywhere between these two meridians, the dioptric power is the same.

Another common form of ametropia, *astigmatism*, is not a spherical refractive error and cannot be fully corrected with a spherical lens. It can be corrected with what is referred to as a *cylindrical lens*. A cylindrical lens has maximum dioptric power in one meridian; the orthogonal (perpendicular) meridian has no dioptric power.

Figure 9-2A shows a glass cylinder fashioned as a cylindrical lens. This cylinder is positioned so that its axis is horizontal. Along the axis, the cylinder is flat—the radius of curvature is infinity—and the lens has no dioptric power. Orthogonal to the horizontal axis, the cylinder has its maximum power (+5.00 D). The power of the other meridians fall somewhere between zero and +5.00 D, with those meridians closest to the +5.00 D meridian manifesting the most dioptric power. The meridians of maximum power and minimum power, which are perpendicular to each other, are called the *principal meridians*. In this example, the meridians whose powers are +5.00 D and zero (i.e., the vertical and horizontal meridians) are the principal meridians.

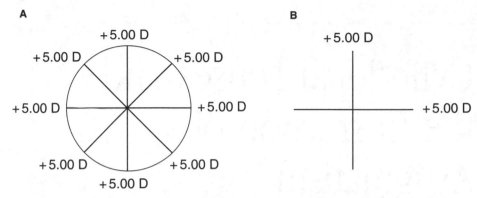

FIGURE 9-1A. A spherical lens has the same power in all of its meridians. **B.** A lens cross for a +5.00 D spherical lens.

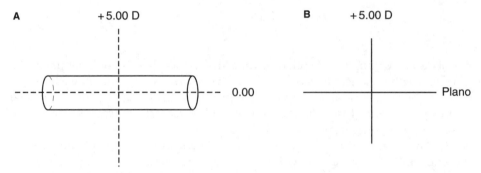

FIGURE 9-2A. This glass cylinder has no power along the horizontal meridian and +5.00 D of power along the vertical meridian. **B.** A lens cross for the cylinder shows the powers in the two principal meridians.

LENS CROSSES

It is customary to represent the powers of a lens's principal meridians on a lens cross. For the lens in Figure 9-2, the horizontal meridian (which is the axis of the lens), has a power of zero and is designated by the term *plano* (abbreviated as *pl*). The vertical meridian is labeled +5.00 D.

Whereas a cylindrical lens has maximum power in one meridian and no power in the orthogonal meridian, a spherical lens has the same power in all meridians. Figure 9-1B shows a lens cross for a +5.00 D spherical lens. Although only two meridians are shown, all other meridians also have a power of +5.00 D.

Corrective lenses frequently combine spherical and cylindrical power. As illustrated in Figure 9-3, a *spherocylindrical lens* can be conceptualized as a combination of a spherical lens and a cylindrical lens. In this case, we have a +2.00 D spherical lens combined with a cylindrical lens that has a maximum power of

+5.00 D and a horizontal axis. The resultant spherocylindrical lens has +7.00 D of power in the vertical meridian and +2.00 D of power in the horizontal meridian. This lens has two focal points. The focal point for the vertical meridian is at +14.29 cm and for the horizontal meridian at +50.00 cm.

By convention, lens meridians (and axes) are specified in degrees measured *counterclockwise* from the 3 o'clock position (Fig. 9-4).[1] Horizontal is always labeled as 180 degrees, not zero degrees. Using this convention, the power of the cylindrical lens in Figure 9-2B is situated at 90 degrees. The axis of this cylindrical lens, which by definition has no power, is 180 degrees. For the spherocylin-

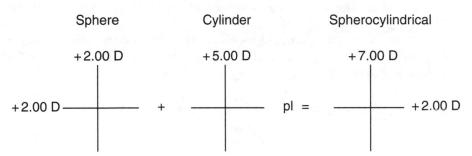

FIGURE 9-3. A spherocylindrical lens can be conceptualized as a combination of a spherical and cylindrical lens.

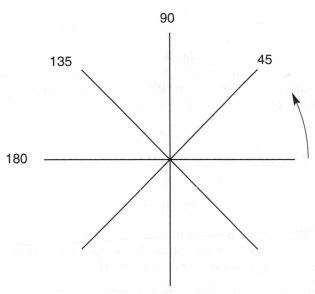

FIGURE 9-4. Lens meridians (and axes) are specified in degrees as measured counterclockwise from the 3 o'clock position. The horizontal should be referred to as 180 degrees—not 0.00 degrees.

[1] When the doctor is facing a patient, the 3 o'clock position is on the doctor's right.

drical lens in Figure 9-3, the 90-degree (vertical) meridian has a power of +7.00 D and the 180-degree (horizontal) meridian has a power of +2.00 D.

LENS FORMULAE/PRESCRIPTIONS

For the sake of clarity, in writing a prescription (formula) for a *spherical* correcting (ophthalmic) lens, it is important to designate the lens power as spherical. This is done with the term *diopters sphere*, which is abbreviated as DS. Sometimes the abbreviations *S* or *Sph*, which stand for *sphere*, are used. Using these conventions, the spherical lens in Figure 9-1 may be labeled as +5.00 DS, +5.00 S or +5.00 Sph.

The formula for a *cylindrical* lens gives (1) the spherical power (which is zero), (2) the cylindrical power, and (3) the axis of the cylinder. For the cylindrical lens in Figure 9-2:

Spherical Power	Cylindrical Power	Axis of the Cylinder
pl	+5.00	180

The lens formula is written as[2]

$$pl = +5.00 \times 180$$

This formula states that: (1) the spherical power is plano (i.e., zero), (2) the cylindrical power is +5.00 D, and (3) the axis of the cylinder is 180 degrees. The maximum power (i.e., +5.00 D) is in the 90-degree meridian.

Now, reconsider the *spherocylindrical* lens in Figure 9-3. Think of this lens as the combination of a spherical lens that has a power of +2.00 DS and a cylindrical lens whose power is pl = +5.00 × 180. The lens formula is

$$+ 2.00 \text{ DS} = + 5.00 \text{ DC} \times 180$$

where *DC* is short for diopters of cylinder.

Or simply

$$+2.00 = +5.00 \times 180$$

This sperocylindrical lens has a power of +7.00 D in the vertical meridian and +2.00 D in the horizontal meridian. Since the cylindrical power is positive, this is referred to as the *plus-cylinder form* of the lens prescription.

---

[2] In this book, we use an equals sign in the lens prescription to represent "combined with." In this case, a plano lens is combined with a +5.00 cylindrical lens that has an axis of 180 degrees.

In Figure 9-5, we have redrawn the lens cross. On the top of the figure, we have broken down the lens into a +2.00 sphere and pl = +5.00 × 180 cylinder (just as we did in Fig. 9-3). On the bottom, we show that there is another way to conceptualize this lens. The lens can be considered as a combination of lenses whose powers are +7.00 DS and pl = –5.00 DC × 090. When conceptualized this way the lens formula is

$$+ 7.00 = -5.00 \times 090$$

This is the *minus-cylinder form* of the prescription.

It is important to keep in mind that the plus- and minus-cylinder forms of the prescription represent the same lens—namely, the spherocylindrical lens in Figure 9-5, which has a power of +7.00 D in the vertical meridian and +2.00 D in the horizontal meridian. **"Plus cylinder form" and "minuscylinder form" are simply different ways of designating the same lens.** Figure 9-6 provides another example. Traditionally, optometrists tend to write

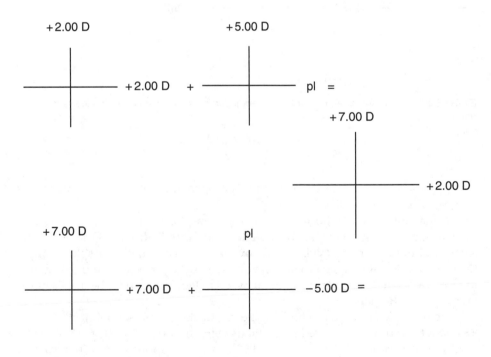

FIGURE 9-5. The spherocylindrical lens on the right can be formed by the combination of either the two lenses on the top (plus-cylinder form) or the two on the bottom (minus-cylinder form).

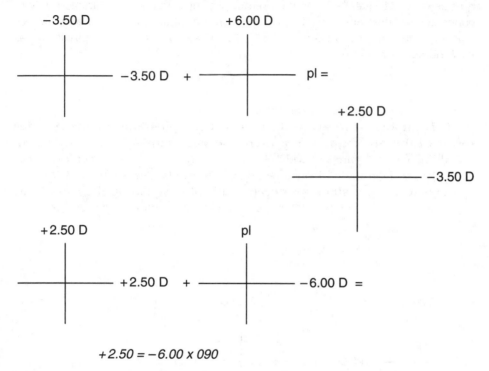

$-3.50 = +6.00 \times 180$

FIGURE 9-6. The plus-cylinder (top) and minus-cylinder forms of the spherocylindrical lens (on the right).

lens prescriptions in minus-cylinder form and ophthalmologists tend to write lens prescriptions in plus-cylinder form.

It is relatively straightforward to *transpose* a plus-cylinder prescription into minus-cylinder form and vice versa. **The rule is as follows:** (1) keeping the signs, add the sphere and cylindrical powers to arrive at the new sphere value, (2) reverse the cylinder sign to arrive at the new cylinder power, and (3) change the axis by 90 degrees to arrive at the new axis. (Remember that the axis is never greater than 180 degrees.)

Let us look at some examples. The plus-cylinder prescription of +2.00 = +5.00 × 180 can be transposed to its minus-cylinder form of +7.00 = −5.00 × 090 (and vice versa). And +2.50 = −6.00 × 090 can be transposed to −3.50 = +6.00 × 180 (and vice versa). These transpositions can be confirmed by drawing lens crosses showing the component lens powers (as in Figs. 9-5 and 9-6).

IMAGE FORMATION: POINT SOURCES

Image formation by spherocylindrical lenses can be confusing. With some persistence, however, you will be able to master this material. The concepts associated with image formation by spherocylindrical lenses have myriad clinical applications, and it is worth the effort to master them.

We begin by briefly reviewing image formation by a spherical lens (Fig. 9-7). Because the lens has the same power in all meridians, the image is located in one plane (i.e., the image plane).

A spherocylindrical lens does not have the same power in all meridians. For instance, the lens in Figure 9-8 has a power of +5.00 D in the vertical meridian and a power of +3.00 D in the horizontal meridian. A point source (the object) located 100 cm in front of the lens is not imaged by this lens in a single plane. The image that is formed by the vertical meridian is focused in one plane and the image focused by the horizontal meridian is located in another plane.

For the purposes of our discussion, we assume that the light rays emitted by a point source diverge either vertically or horizontally.[3] First, consider the image formed by the vertical meridian, which is the stronger meridian of the lens (Fig. 9-8). The vertical meridian focuses those rays that diverge vertically from the object. These rays, which are said to have vertical divergence, are focused by the vertical meridian at a plane that is +25.00 cm from the lens. If you place a screen at this plane, however, there is not a point but rather a thin horizontal line. This line is formed because the horizontally diverging object rays are focused by the horizontal meridian at +50.00 cm, not at 25.00 cm.

The upper and lower edges of the horizontal image are sharply focused because they are they are formed by the in-focus vertical meridian (Fig. 9-8). If the lens were spherical, we would have a point image. But because the horizontal meridian has a different power, the image is smeared in a horizontal dimension (and has blurred left and right edges).

Now, consider the image formed by the weaker horizontal meridian. This meridian focuses rays that have horizontal divergence—rays that diverge from the object in the horizontal dimension. These horizontally diverging rays are focused by the horizontal meridian at a plane that is +50.00 cm from the lens. At this plane, however, there is not a point but a vertical line. This is because

---

[3] Spread your fingers apart and place your palms together such that the fingers of your two hands are facing each other. Now, rotate your hands so that your palms are horizontal. Next, keep your wrists together while separating your hands. Think of your fingers as vertically diverging light rays. To illustrate horizontally diverging light rays, keep your wrists together and rotate your palms so that they are vertical. When your (vertical) palms are separated (but your wrists are together), you can think of your fingers as horizontally diverging light rays.

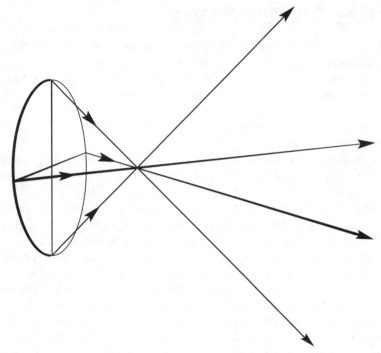

FIGURE 9-7. A spherical lens focuses a point source in one image plane.

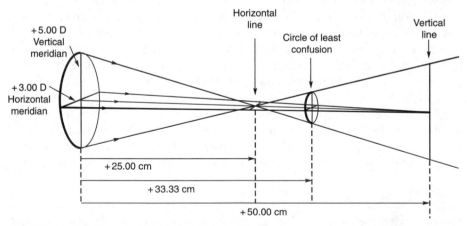

FIGURE 9-8. A spherocylindrical lens (which has a power of +5.00 D in the vertical meridian and +3.00 D in the horizontal meridian) focuses a point source in two image planes. The object distance is −100.00 cm. See text for further details.

the vertically diverging object rays are focused by the vertical meridian at +25.00 cm; beyond +25.00 cm, these rays diverge, forming a vertical smear at 50.00 cm.

The left and right edges of the vertical line are in sharp focus at 50.00 cm because they are formed by the in-focus horizontal meridian of the lens. The image is, however, smeared in the vertical dimension (and has blurred upper and lower edges) because the vertical meridian is in focus at 25.00 cm, not 50.00 cm.

If we place a screen directly behind the lens and move it away from the lens, we will see that a horizontal line is found at +25.00 cm and a vertical line at +50.00 cm. The interval that is bracketed by these two images is referred to as the *interval of Sturm*. Within this interval, we find a circle at +33.33 cm from the lens. This circle—called the *circle of least confusion*—is located at the plane where the vertical and horizontal meridians are equally defocused.

The circle of least confusion is *not* linearly centered between the planes of focus of the two principal meridians, but **centered dioptrically**. For the point source located 100.00 cm in front of the lens (Fig. 9-8), the *dioptric* location of the circle of least confusion is calculated as

$$+2.00 \text{ D} + [(4.00 \text{ D} - 2.00 \text{ D})/2] = +3.00 \text{ D}$$

Therefore, the *linear* location is

$$(1.00) \ (100)/+3.00 \text{ D} = +33.33 \text{ cm}$$

The circle of least confusion is located 33.33 cm to the right of the lens.

IMAGE FORMATION: EXTENDED SOURCES

An extended source, such as the cross in Figure 9-9, is formed by an infinite number of point sources. *Assume that this cross serves as an object for a spherocylindrical lens that has a power of +5.00 D in the vertical meridian and +3.00 D in the horizontal meridian. The object distance is 100.00 cm. Locate the images and draw these images.*

First, consider the horizontal line of the object. The points that constitute this line emit light rays with vertical and horizontal divergence. The rays with vertical divergence are focused by the vertical meridian to form a horizontal line at +25.00 cm.

The vertical line of the object is also made up of points that emit vertically and horizontally diverging rays. Those rays with horizontal divergence are focused by the horizontal meridian at +50.00 cm to form a vertical line.

Figure 9-9 shows the images produced by the lens. At +25.00 cm, we have a focused horizontal line and a blurred vertical line. The focused horizontal line is an image of the horizontal line of the cross. The upper and lower edges of this line are sharply focused. The object rays with vertical divergence are focused by the vertical meridian to form these focused edges. In comparison,

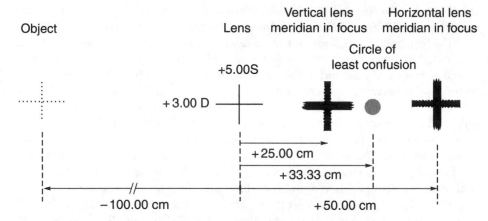

FIGURE 9-9. A spherocylindrical lens focuses an extended object in two planes. See text for further details.

the left and right edges are blurred. Horizontally diverging rays emitted by the horizontal line, which are focused at +50.00 cm, form these fuzzy edges.

At +25.00 cm, there is also a blurred vertical line. This is the blurred image of the vertical line of the cross. The horizontally diverging rays emitted by the vertical line are focused by the horizontal meridian at +50.00 cm, not at 25.00 cm. The rays that form the vertical line at +25.00 cm are smeared horizontally because the horizontal meridian is not in focus at this distance.

Now consider image formation in the plane that is +50.00 cm from the lens. The vertical line's horizontally diverging rays are focused by the horizontal meridian of the lens to form a vertical line with sharply focused left and right edges. In comparison, the upper and lower borders of this line are blurred. The vertical line's vertically diverging rays, which are focused by the vertical meridian at 25.00 cm, form these blurred upper and lower edges.

There is also a blurred horizontal line at +50.00 cm. The blurring (or smearing) is in a vertical direction because the vertical meridian, which focuses the vertically diverging rays emitted by the horizontal line, is in focus at 25.00 cm, not 50.00 cm.

Where is the circle of confusion for this extended object? As is the case for a point source, the circle is dioptrically centered between the focused images of the two principal meridians (i.e., where the defocus of the vertical meridian is equal to the defocus of the horizontal meridian).

Let us summarize a few key points on image formation by spherocylindrical lenses[4]:

---

[4] It is easiest to understand this material if you think of a lens that has positive power in both of its meridians.

1. A point source (i.e., point object) emits rays that diverge vertically and rays that diverge horizontally.
2. The vertically diverging object rays are focused by the vertical meridian. A horizontal line is formed in the image plane of the vertical meridian.
3. The horizontally diverging object rays are focused by the horizontal meridian. A vertical line is formed in the image plane of the horizontal meridian.
4. The vertically diverging rays emitted by a horizontal line (object) are focused by the vertical meridian as a horizontal line.
5. The horizontally diverging rays emitted by a vertical line are focused by the horizontal meridian as a vertical line.

This material can be difficult to conceptualize, so do not worry if you are finding it confusing. Take a break—maybe sleep on it—and then reread the section on image formation (for both point and extended sources). It will click.

ASTIGMATISM: DEFINITIONS AND CLASSIFICATIONS

The power of an *astigmatic eye* is spherocylindrical[5]. In *regular astigmatism*, the two principal meridians of the eye are perpendicular to each other. This form of astigmatism, which is by far the more common form, can be corrected with spherocylindrical lenses. *Irregular astigmatism* is generally secondary to trauma, surgery, or a disease process. The principal meridians are not perpendicular to each other, and the eye cannot be corrected with a spherocylindrical lens.

When an astigmatic eye[6] images a point source, the image is similar to that formed by a spherocylindrical lens. Astigmatism is classified according to the location of the image with respect to the retina (with accommodation relaxed). Figure 9-10 shows image formation in the various forms of astigmatism.

In addition to classifying astigmatism based on image location, it is common to classify it according to the meridian of the eye that has the most converging refracting power. If the vertical meridian *of the eye*[7] is strongest, we call the astigmatism *with-the-rule*. *Against-the-rule* is present when the horizontal meridian *of the eye* is strongest. When the strongest meridian *of the eye* is neither vertical nor horizontal but falls somewhere between the two (e.g., 135 +/− 15° or 45 +/− 15°), we have *oblique astigmatism*.

Consider an eye that requires the following lens to obtain the best corrected acuity (e.g., 20/20):

---

[5] The Greek term *stigma* refers to a point or small mark. Astigmatism refers to an image that is not a point.
[6] Unless otherwise specified, assume that the term *astigmatism* refers to the power of the eye, not the correction.
[7] The phrase "of the eye" is italicized to emphasize that we are referring to the power of the eye, not the correction.

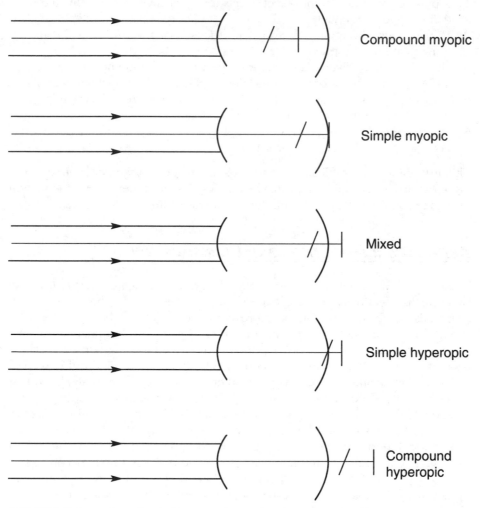

FIGURE 9-10. Image formation in the various forms of ocular astigmatism. (Assume that the object is a point source located at infinity.)

$$-5.00 = -2.00 \times 180$$

Classify this eye's astigmatism. It is important to keep in mind that this lens is used to *correct* the eye's astigmatism. Figure 9-11A shows that the eye has compound myopic astigmatism—both optical meridians are focused in front of the retina. For the image to be focused on the retina, the vertical meridian of the eye requires a correction of –7.00 D of power and the horizontal meridian requires –5.00 D. Since the vertical meridian requires more minus power, it is the stronger of the two meridians: the patient has with-the-rule compound myopic astigmatism. *Let us take another example. The correcting lens is as follows:*

$$+2.00 - -3.00 \times 090$$

The correction for the vertical meridian is +2.00 D and for the horizontal meridian it is −1.00 D. This is a case of mixed astigmatism because one meridian is focused in front of the retina (the horizontal meridian) and the other is focused behind the retina (the vertical meridian) (Fig. 9-11B). Since the horizontal meridian has the greater converging power, the eye has against-the-rule mixed astigmatism.

At birth, human neonates generally have 0.75 to 2.00 DC of astigmatism. The axis of the astigmatism is apparently influenced by the neonate's race, with Chinese infants tending to have with-the-rule astigmatism and Caucasian infants tending to have against-the-rule astigmatism (Thorn et al., 1987). This early astigmatism tends to decrease as the infant progresses through early childhood (Gwiazda et al., 1984).

As adults age, the axis of the astigmatism tends to become more against-the-rule. This is apparently due to aging of the crystalline lens.

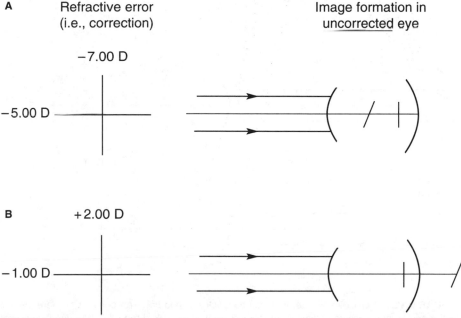

FIGURE 9-11A. Image formation in with-the-rule compound myopic astigmatism. **B.** Image formation in against-the-rule mixed astigmatism. (Assume that the object is a point source located at infinity.)

JACKSON CROSSED-CYLINDER TEST

The *Jackson crossed-cylinder (JCC)* test is the most frequently used subjective clinical procedure to determine the amount of a patient's astigmatism. Figure 9-12A shows a crossed-cylinder lens. The power in one of the principal meridians of a crossed cylinder is equal and opposite to the power in the other principal meridian (e.g., one meridian has a power of +0.25 D and the other meridian has a power of −0.25 D). The crossed cylinder is mounted in front of the patient's eye such that it can be quickly flipped between the position where the vertical meridian has plus power and the position where it has minus power.

How can the crossed cylinder be used to determine the amount of astigmatism? Figure 9-12B shows the position of the retinal images formed when an

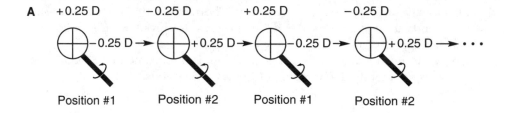

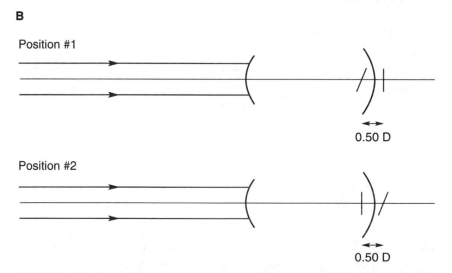

FIGURE 9-12A. A crossed-cylinder lens can be quickly flipped between position 1 where the vertical meridian has positive power and position 2 where the vertical meridian has negative power. To flip the crossed cylinder, the stem is twisted between the thumb and forefinger. **B.** Image formation in an emmetropic eye when looking through a crossed-cylinder lens in position 1 (top) and position 2 (bottom). Note that the sequence of the (line) images reverses when the crossed cylinder is flipped.

emmetrope views a distant object through a crossed cylinder. The circle of least confusion is located on the retina. When the crossed cylinder is flipped, the sequence of the line images reverses but the amount of astigmatism remains the same (i.e., 0.50 DC) and the circle of least confusion remains on the retina. Consequently, the patient will report that the image is equally blurred for both positions of the crossed cylinder.

Now consider the astigmatic eye in Figure 9-13A, which has a power of +62.00 D in the vertical meridian and +58.00 D in the horizontal meridian (with-the-rule mixed astigmatism). When a crossed-cylinder lens is placed in front of the eye so that its positive meridian is oriented vertically (position 1), the amount of astigmatism is 4.50 D (i.e., 62.25 D – 57.75 D = 4.50 D). When the crossed cylinder is flipped so that its vertical meridian now has negative power (position 2), the amount of astigmatism is 3.50 D (i.e., 61.75 – 58.25 = 3.50 D). When given a choice, the patient will say that position 2 is clearer that position 1. This is because the amount of astigmatism is less in position 2. The doctor can then add minus power to the vertical meridian (i.e., minus cylinder with an *axis* of 180 degrees) and repeat the crossed-cylinder test until the patient reports that the image is equally blurred in positions 1 and 2. (As discussed in the next section, during crossed-cylinder testing, the doctor adds plus spherical power to keep the circle of least confusion positioned on the retina.) If the doctor adds too much minus power to the vertical meridian, the patient will report that position 1 now is clearer that position 2. The astigmatism is corrected when the images are equally blurred, the situation depicted in Figure 9-13B.

SPHERICAL EQUIVALENCY

Consider the astigmatic eye in Figure 9-14. Assume that the vertical meridian has a power of 60.00 D and is focused on the retina. The prescription is

$$plano = +5.00 \times 090$$

Suppose that you do not have access to cylindrical or spherocylindrical lenses and can prescribe only a spherical lens to correct this eye. What would be the best spherical lens to prescribe?

To minimize the amount of blur that the patient experiences, the circle of least confusion should be centered on the retina. This may be accomplished by prescribing a so-called *spherical equivalent* lens. This spherical lens has a power equal to the sum of the sphere power and one-half of the cylinder power. In the above case, the spherical equivalent is +2.50 DS (Fig. 9-14).

For the JCC test to produce accurate results, the circle of least confusion must remain on the retina. For each –0.50 of cylindrical power that is added during the testing procedure, the spherical equivalent power changes by –0.25 DS. That is, if the circle of least confusion falls on the retina, the addition of –0.50 DC will cause the circle to fall –0.25 DS behind the retina. To keep the circle of

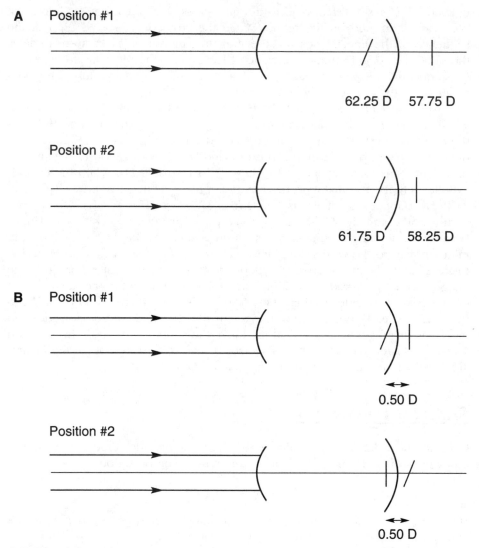

A Position #1

62.25 D   57.75 D

Position #2

61.75 D   58.25 D

B Position #1

0.50 D

Position #2

0.50 D

FIGURE 9-13A. Image formation in an uncorrected astigmatic eye when looking through a crossed-cylinder lens (see Fig. 9-12) in position 1 and position 2. **B.** After correction of the astigmatism (and any spherical refractive error), the amount of image blur is the same whether the crossed-cylinder lens is in position 1 or position 2. Note that the sequence of the (line) images reverses when the crossed cylinder is flipped.

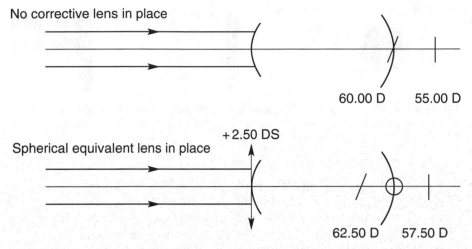

FIGURE 9-14. A spherical equivalent lens centers the interval of Sturm dioptically (not linearly) on the retina. As such, the circle of least confusion falls upon the retina. In this figure, the spherical equivalent is +2.50 D (bottom).

least confusion on the retina during the JCC test, the doctor can increase the spherical power by +0.25 DS each time he or she increases the cylinder power by −0.50 DC.

WHAT DOES THE ASTIGMAT SEE?

A patient with uncorrected myopia or uncompensated hyperopia experiences uniform blur—the image is equally blurred in all directions: up and down, left and right, and every direction in between. For example, when an uncorrected myope views a point source, he or she perceives a blurred circle (Fig. 9-15A). *What does the following uncorrected astigmat perceive when viewing a point source?*

$$pl = -2.00 \times 180$$

This patient has with-the-rule simple myopic astigmatism. The horizontal meridian of the eye requires no correction. This meridian focuses the object's horizontally diverging rays onto the retina. Now consider the stronger vertical meridian. This meridian focuses the vertically diverging rays as a point in front of the retina. After forming this image, these rays diverge vertically and fall upon the retina to form a vertical line. Since the rays are diverging vertically when they strike the retina, the upper and lower borders of the line are blurred (or smeared). The patient reports seeing a vertical line with sharp lateral edges and fuzzy vertical edges (Fig. 9-15B).

FIGURE 9-15A. Appearance of a point source to an uncorrected myope. **B.** Appearance of a point source to an uncorrected with-the-rule simple myopic astigmat. **C.** Appearance of the optotype **F** to an uncorrected with-the-rule simple myopic astigmat.

Suppose we ask this patient to read a visual acuity chart. *Are there any optotypes[8] that the patient will find particularly difficult to resolve?* Consider the **F** optotype. To correctly identify this optotype (which is an extended object), it is necessary to resolve the gap between the two horizontal line segments. These horizontal lines are refracted by the vertical meridian to form horizontal lines that are focused in front of the retina. The rays then diverge vertically to form horizontal line on the retina that are vertically smeared. As with the point source, the blur is vertical (Fig. 9-15C). As a result, the gap is difficult to see. Patients with this type of refractive error often mistakenly identify an **F** as a **P**.

This astigmat will have less difficulty identifying the vertical line in the **F**. The horizontal meridian of the eye focuses the vertical line on the retina. Its lateral edges will be sharply focused, but its vertical edges will be smeared because they are formed by the out-of-focus vertical meridian.

BIBLIOGRAPHY

Gwiazda J, Scheiman M, Mohindra I, Held R. Astigmatism in infants: Changes in axis and amount from birth to six years. *Invest Ophthalmol Vis Sci.* 1984;25:88.

Thorn F, Held R, Fang L. Orthogonal astigmatic axis in Chinese and Caucasian infants. *Invest Ophthalmol Vis Sci.* 1987;28:191.

---

[8] The figures on a visual acuity chart—letters or other symbols designed with the intent of measuring visual acuity—are called *optotypes.*

P Self-Assessment Problems

1. A lens has the following formula: −2.00 = +1.00 × 180. (a) Draw a lens cross. (b) Write the prescription in minus-cylinder form.

2. A point source is located 50.00 cm in front of the following lens: +4.00 = +2.00 × 180. (a) Which meridian is focused closest to the lens? (b) Is the line that is focused closest to the lens horizontal or vertical? (c) How far is this image located from the lens? (d) Answer questions *b* and *c* for the image that is located furthest from the lens (i.e., the image formed by the other meridian of the lens). (e) Calculate the linear extent of the interval of Sturm. (f) Locate the circle of least confusion.

3. A point source is located 25.00 cm in front of the following lens: +7.00 = −2.00 × 180. Answer all the questions asked for Problem 2.

4. A cross is located 40.00 cm in front of the following lens: +5.00 = +1.00 × 180. (a) At what distance is the horizontal line imaged? (b) At what distance is the vertical line imaged? (c) What is the linear extent of the interval of Sturm? (d) Locate the circle of least confusion.

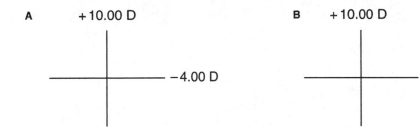

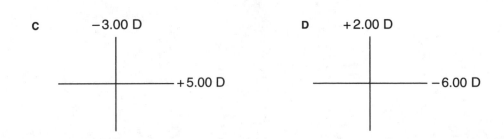

5. A cross is situated 40.00 cm in front of the following lens: +6.00 = −2.00 × 180. Answer all the questions asked for Problem 4.

6. Consider the following lens crosses:

Write the lens prescriptions in both minus-cylinder and plus-cylinder form.

7. A patient's refractive error is corrected with the following lens: +4.00 = −3.00 × 090. (a) Is the patient's astigmatism with-the-rule or against-the-rule? What form of astigmatism does the patient have (see Fig. 9-10)? (b) Answer the same questions for a prescription of −1.00 = −2.00 × 180. (c) Answer the same questions for a prescription of −3.00 = +4.00 × 090.

8. A patient compares a grating consisting of horizontal bars to a grating consisting of vertical bars. He reports that both gratings' bars appear blurry, with the vertical bars appearing clearer than the horizontal bars. (a) Is the patient more likely to have with-the-rule or against-the-rule myopic astigmatism? (b) Justify you answer.

Prisms

10

A prism refracts light and changes its direction. Prisms do not affect the vergence of light because their surfaces are flat: the surfaces have no dioptric power.[1]

Figure 10-1 shows the refraction that occurs at the two surfaces of a prism. The refraction at each surface is predictable from Snell's law. For this prism (and all ophthalmic prisms), **light rays are deviated toward the base of the prism**. When an observer views an object through the prism, he or she sees an image of the object. **The image is displaced toward the apex of the prism**. This image is virtual.

ANGLE OF DEVIATION

Figure 10-2 shows the path of a light ray traveling through a prism whose *apical (or refracting) angle* is α. At the first surface, the ray has an angle of incidence of θ_1, an angle of refraction of θ_1', and an *angle of deviation*[2] of β_1. The angle of incidence at the second surface is θ_2, the angle of refraction is θ_2', and the angle of deviation is β_2. The *total angle of deviation* is β. From the geometry, we can see that

$$\alpha = \theta'_1 + \theta_2$$
$$\beta = \beta_1 + \beta_2$$
$$\beta = \theta_1 + \theta'_2 - \alpha$$

Let us do a problem. *A crown glass prism has an apical angle of 60.0 degrees. The angle of incidence at the first surface is 50.0 degrees. By how many degrees does the prism deviate the incident light?* At the first surface we apply Snell's law:

---

[1] For a flat surface, the radius of curvature is infinity.

[2] Recall that for Snell's law, the angles of incidence and refraction are defined with respect to the normal to the surface. In comparison, the angle of deviation is defined with respect to the direction of the incident ray.

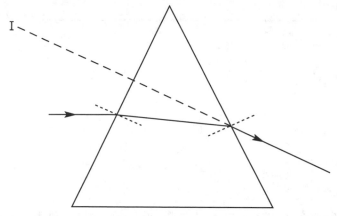

FIGURE 10-1. A prism refracts light and changes its direction. The location of the virtual image is represented by *I*.

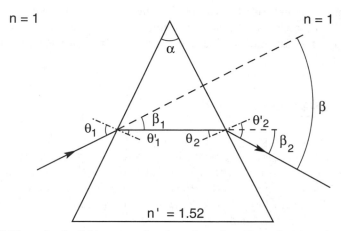

FIGURE 10-2. The path of a light ray traveling through a prism. The apical (or refracting) angle is represented by α, the angle of deviation at the first surface by β_1, the angle of deviation at the second surface by β_2, and the total angle of deviation by β. See text for further details.

$$n \sin \theta_1 = n' \sin \theta'_1$$
$$(1.00)(\sin 50.0°) = (1.52)(\sin \theta'_1)$$
$$\theta'_1 = 30.3°$$

We now calculate θ_2:

$$\alpha = \theta'_1 + \theta_2$$
$$60.0° = 30.3° + \theta_2$$
$$\theta_2 = 29.7°$$

At the second surface we have

$$n' \sin \theta_2 = n \sin \theta'_2$$
$$(1.52)(\sin 29.7°) = (1.00)(\sin \theta'_2)$$
$$\theta'_2 = 48.9°$$

We now calculate β:

$$\beta = \theta_1 + \theta'_2 - \alpha$$
$$\beta = 50.0° + 48.9° - 60°$$
$$\beta = 38.9°$$

The total angle of deviation is 38.9 degrees.

The total angle of deviation can also be determined by summing the deviations produced by each surface. The deviation produced by the first surfaces is

$$\beta_1 = 50.0° - 30.3° = 19.7°$$

And the deviation produced by the second surface is

$$\beta_2 = 48.9° - 29.7° = 19.2°$$

The total deviation is

$$\beta = \beta_1 + \beta_2$$
$$\beta = 19.7° + 19.2°$$
$$\beta = 38.9°$$

PRISM POWER

Figure 10-3A shows a light ray that, after refraction by a prism, falls upon a screen that is at a distance of 1.00 m. The light ray is deviated 1.00 cm from its original destination. **A prism that deviates a light ray 1.00 cm at a distance of 1.00 m is said to have a power of 1 *prism diopter*** (abbreviated pd or denoted by the symbol $^\Delta$). If the ray is deviated 5.00 cm at a distance of 1.00 m, the power of the prism is 5^Δ. Likewise, a prism that deviates a ray of light 8.00 cm at a distance of 400.00 cm has a power of 2^Δ.

We can more formally define a prism's power with the following formulae:

$$P_p = (100)(\tan \sigma)$$

or

$$\boldsymbol{P_p = (100)(x/d)}$$

where

P_p = the prism power in prism diopters
x = the distance that the light ray is deviated
d = the distance at which the deviation is measured (Fig. 10-3B)

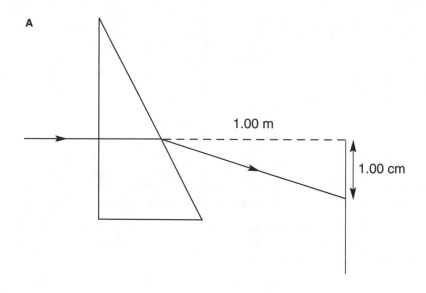

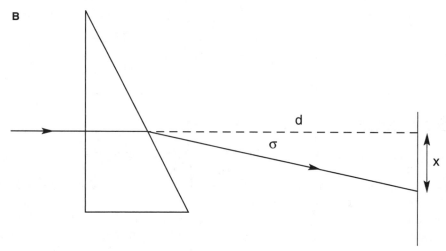

FIGURE 10-3A. A prism that deviates a light ray 1.00 cm at a distance of 1.00 m has a power of 1 prism diopter. **B.** Distances pertinent to defining a prism diopter. See text for further details.

For instance, if a prism deviates a light ray 8.00 cm at a distance of 400.00 cm, its power is calculated as follows:

$$P_{\text{p}} = (100)(\tan \sigma)$$
$$P_{\text{p}} = (100)\ (8 \text{ cm}/400 \text{ cm})$$
$$P_{\text{p}} = 2^{\Delta}$$

PRISMATIC EFFECTS OF LENSES

A lens can be thought of as consisting of two prisms (Fig. 10-4). The prismatic power increases as the distance from the optical center of the lens and/or the lens power increases (Fig. 10-5).[3] The greater the prism power, the more the image is displaced (Fig. 10-6). There is no prismatic power along the optical axis of a lens—a light ray that travels along the optical axis is not deviated.

Keep in mind that a lens has both dioptric power and prism power. The dioptric power, which is due to the curvature of the lens surfaces, is manifest as a change in the vergence of the light rays. The prismatic power is manifest as a displacement of the image toward the apex of the prism.

PRENTICE'S RULE

Figure 10-7 shows how the prismatic power of a lens can be quantifed. A light ray from a distant object is focused at a plus lens's secondary focal point. The distances are in centimeters. We see that

$$P_p = (100)(d/f')$$

but

$$f' = 100/P$$

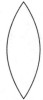 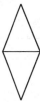

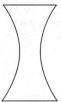 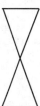

FIGURE 10-4. Lenses (left) can be conceptualized as combinations of two prisms (right).

---

[3]Consider the optical center of a lens to be the intersection of the lens and the optical axis.

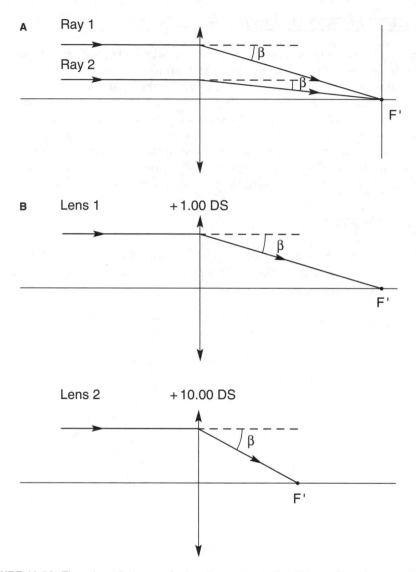

FIGURE 10-5A. The prismatic power of a lens increases as the distance from the optical center increases (i.e., ray 1 is more deviated than ray 2). The optical center of a thin lens is the intersection of the lens and the optical axis. **B.** A lens's prismatic power increases as the dioptric power of the lens increases.

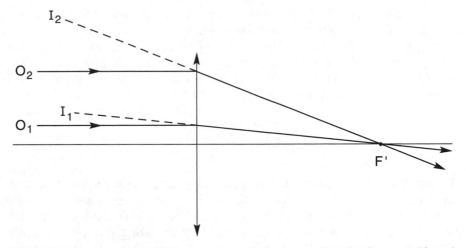

FIGURE 10-6. When an object (O_2) is viewed through a point on a lens that is removed from the optical axis, the image (I_2) appears more displaced than when an object (O_1) is viewed through a point close to the optical axis. In the extreme case, an object that is viewed along the optical axis of a lens does not appear displaced.

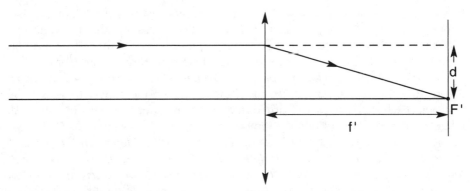

FIGURE 10-7. Distances pertinent to Prentice's rule. All distances are in centimeters. See text for further details.

therefore

$$P_p = (d)(P)$$

where

      d = the distance in centimeters between the optical center and the point at which the ray is incident upon the lens

      P = the dioptric power of the lens

Since d must be in centimeters, the formula is often expressed as

$$P_p = (d_{cm})(P)$$

This handy relationship, which allows us to calculate the prismatic power of an ophthalmic lens, is referred to as *Prentice's rule*.

A patient's right ophthalmic lens is decentered so that the patient looks through a point 2.0 mm temporal to its optical center (Fig. 10-8A). If the dioptric power of the lens is +6.00 DS, what is the prismatic effect? We use Prentice's rule to determine the prism power:

$$P_p = (d_{cm})(P)$$
$$P_p = (0.20\ cm)(6.00\ D)$$
$$P_p = 1.2\ ^\Delta$$

The prismatic power is $1.2\ ^\Delta$ *base-in* when the patient looks through a point 2.0 mm temporal to the optical axis. The prism power is designated as base-in because the base of the prism is facing toward the patient's midline. If the lens were −6.00 DS, the prismatic power would be 1.2^Δ *base-out* because the base of the prism is temporal (Fig. 10-8B).

CLINICAL APPLICATIONS

In viewing the object in Figure 10-8A, the patient must turn her right eye in a temporal direction for the image to fall on the fovea (assume that the other eye is occluded). Prisms have important clinical applications because of their ability to displace an image in a direction that benefits visual function and/or comfort.

Consider a patient with exophoria—a tendency for the eyes to turn outward. Figure 10-9 shows that base-in prisms allow the exophoric patient to view a distant object while her eyes are turned in an outward direction. This may provide relief for asthenopic and other symptoms.

An exophoric patient is fully corrected with −4.00 DS lenses in the spectacle plane. The patient requires a prescription of 2.0^Δ base-in prism to alleviate symptoms of near asthenopia. Her interpupillary distance (abbreviated as ipd) is 56 mm when viewing near objects.[4] *How can we incorporate the prism correction into the −4.00 D lenses?*

It is common clinical practice to divide the prismatic correction between the two eyes equally. Where must the patient look through a −4.00 DS lens to obtain $1.0\ ^\Delta$ base-in? Prentice's rule is very helpful in cases like this:

$$P_p = (d_{cm})(P)$$
$$1.0^\Delta = d_{cm}\ (4.00D)$$
$$d = 0.25\ cm, \text{ or } 2.5\ mm$$

---

[4] The interpupillary distance is the distance between the centers of a patient's pupils.

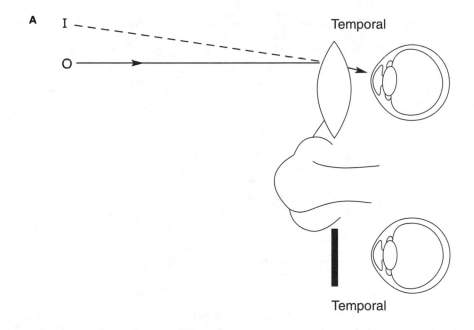

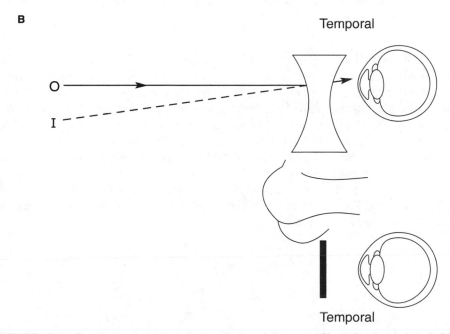

FIGURE 10-8A. Prentice's rule can be used to calculate the amount of base-in prism induced when a patient looks through a point that is temporal to the optical axis of a plus lens. You are looking-down upon the patient's head. The left eye is occluded. **B.** Likewise, Prentice's rule can be used to calculate the amount of base-out prism induced when a patient looks through a point that is temporal to the optical axis of a minus lens.

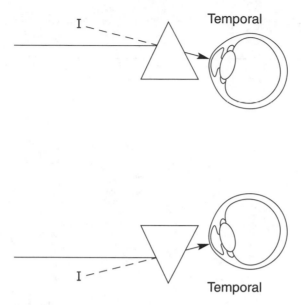

FIGURE 10-9. In viewing a distant object, this patient's eyes have a tendency to turn outward (i.e., the patient is exophoric). The base-in prisms displace the images temporally, thereby allowing the patient's eyes to turn outward while viewing a distant object. (You are looking down upon the patient's head.)

If the patient looks through a point 2.5 mm nasal to the lens's optical axis, he experiences 1.0^{Δ} base-in. This occurs when the lens is made such that its optical center is 2.5 mm temporal to the center of the patient's pupil (Fig. 10-10). If, instead of placing the optical axis of the lens at a distance of 28 mm from the patient's midline (56 mm / 2 = 28 mm), it is placed 30.5 mm from the midline (28.0 mm + 2.5 mm = 30.5 mm), the patient experiences 1.0^{Δ} base-in.

To obtain a total prismatic effect of 2.0^{Δ}, the optical center of each lens must be displaced 2.5 mm temporally. When wearing 4.00 D lenses, whose optical centers are separated by 61 mm, the patient receives the benefit of 2.0^{Δ} base-in prism (at near). The prism power allows the eyes to point in a more comfortable outward (exophoric) direction.

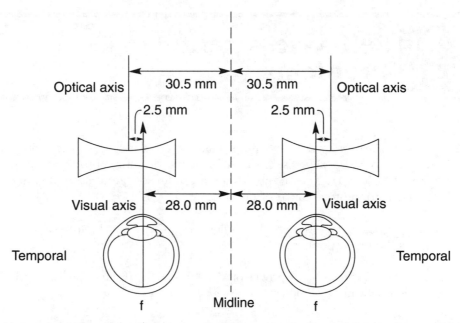

FIGURE 10-10. A total of 2.0$^\Delta$ base-in prism will be included in a spectacle prescription of –4.00 DS OU if each eye looks through a point 2.5 mm nasal to the optical axis. The visual axis intersects the fovea, *f*. (You are looking down upon the patient's head.)

P Self-Assessment Problems

1. A crown glass prism has an apical angle of 60.00 degrees. The angle of incidence is 30.00 degrees. (a) Determine the deviation produced by the first surface. (b) Determine the deviation produced by the second surface. (c) Calculate the total angle of deviation.

2. A crown glass prism deviates a ray of light by 4.00 cm at a distance of 5.00 m. What is the prism power?

3. A crown glass prism has a power of 15.00^Δ. At what distance will the prism deviate a light ray by 2.00 cm?

4. What is the prismatic power at a distance of 5.00 mm from the optical center of a +8.00 D plastic lens?

5. A crown glass lens has a power of –6.00 D. To obtain a prism power of 2.00^Δ, the patient would have to look through a point that is how far from the center of the lens?

6. An object is located 13.00 cm in front of a crown glass prism that has a refracting angle of 65.00 degrees. What is the vergence of the rays that emerge from the prism? (Assume that the prism has no thickness.)

7. A crown glass prism has an apical angle of 84.0 degrees. The angle of incidence is 45.0 degrees. (a) With respect to the normal, at what angle does the ray emerge from the prism? (b) What phenomenon is taking place?

Depth of Field

11

An object that is conjugate with the retina is by definition focused on the retina. If the object is a point, then the image is a point. Figure 11-1A shows a myopic eye that has no ability to accommodate (i.e., the eye of an *absolute presbyope*). Point Y is imaged onto the retina at Y′. For an object that is closer to the eye— say at Z—the imaged is focused behind the retina at Z′. The blurred retinal image is called a *blur circle*. A similar effect occurs for an object at X: the image is focused at X′ and a blur circle is formed on the retina. Figure 11-1B shows how these blur circles may appear to the observer.

The size of the blur circle depends on the amount of defocus and the diameter of the pupil. The more the object is out of focus, the larger the blur circle (Fig. 11-2A). As Figure 11-2B shows, the smaller the pupil, the smaller the retinal blur circle.

BLUR CIRCLES AND VISUAL ACUITY

Consider an uncorrected 1.00 D myope who observes the optotype **E** on a visual acuity chart that is located 20 ft away (optical infinity). The optotype can be thought of as an infinite number of point sources (Fig. 11-3A). Since this eye is not in focus, each of the point sources forms a blur circle on the retina. As a result, the image of the optotype is defocused. Depending on the size of the optotype and the diameter of the patient's pupil, the patient may see a blurry **E** or may not recognize the optoype because she cannot resolve the gaps between the horizontal lines of the optotype.

Suppose we ask the uncorrected 1.00 D myope to view the eye chart through a small aperture, referred to as a *pinhole*. If the pinhole is smaller than the patient's pupil (i.e., it is an *artificial pupil*), it reduces the size of all the blur circles that constitute the **E**. As a result, the patient is better able to resolve this and other optotypes on the acuity chart (Fig. 11-3B).

An isolated pinhole (or a cluster of pinholes) is an important clinical tool (Fig. 11-4). When a patient's acuity is reduced due to optical blur, as in the case of ametropia, viewing though a pinhole will typically improve the visual acuity.

A

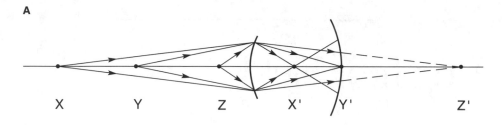

X   Y   Z   X'   Y'   Z'

B

Point X   Point Y   Point Z

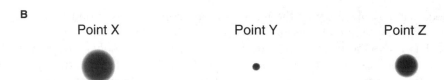

FIGURE 11-1A. Point source Y is imaged on the retina, while point sources X and Z are out of focus and form blur circles on the retina. **B.** Appearance of a point source that is in focus (Y) and point sources that are out of focus (X and Z).

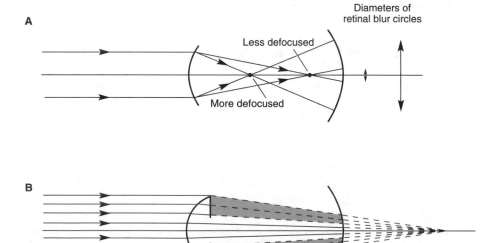

Diameters of
retinal blur circles

A

Less defocused

More defocused

B

FIGURE 11-2A. As the amount of defocus increases, the diameter of the retinal blur circle also increases. **B.** Decreasing the size of the pupil reduces the diameter of the retinal blur circle. In this diagram, the light rays in the shaded area do not reach the retina because the pupil blocks them; consequently, the diameter of the retinal blur circle is decreased.

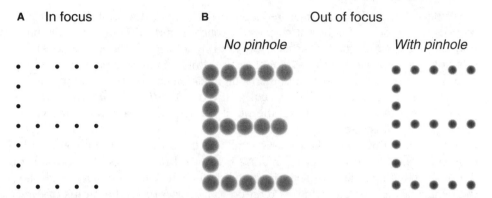

FIGURE 11-3A. An optotype (or any extended object) is made up of point sources. **B.** If the point sources that constitute the optotype are defocused, the optotype itself appears defocused. A pinhole decreases the diameters of the blur circles, thereby increasing the resolvability of the optotype.

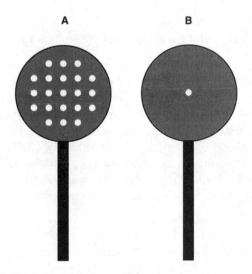

FIGURE 11-4. In the clinic, it is generally more efficient to use a cluster of pinholes (as in **A**) rather than have the patient search for a single pinhole (illustrated in **B**).

Consider the patient who has a distance visual acuity of 20/40, but improves to 20/20 when viewing through a pinhole. In such a case, it is highly likely that the reduced visual acuity is due to a refractive error. If the pinhole does not improve visual acuity, you must suspect another etiology (such as disease).

As we age, our pupil becomes smaller. In elderly people, the pupil can be rather small—a condition referred to as *senile miosis*. There are some advantages to this condition. In uncorrected (or undercorrected) ametropia and presbyopia, the small pupil may improve visual acuity through the *pinhole effect*.

While the smaller pupil may reduce the diameter of the blur circles, it also reduces the amount of light that reaches the retina. A reduction in retinal illumination may cause a reduction in visual acuity (for physiologic, not optical reasons) that offsets improvements due to the pinhole effect. Bright lighting conditions can help to compensate for the reduction in retinal illumination caused by senile miosis.

A small pupil can also limit visual acuity due to *diffraction*, which occurs when the wavelength of light and the pupil diameter approach the same value. Figure 11-5A illustrates the *diffraction pattern* (i.e., the distribution of light) found on the retina when the pupil is small and the object is a point source. The diffraction pattern consists of alternating bright and dark rings. The portion of the pattern that includes the peak (i.e., the bright center) and the first trough (i.e., the center of the first dark ring) is referred to as *Airy's disk*. The radius of Airy's disk (θ) in radians is given by the following formula:

$$\theta = 1.22\lambda/d$$

where

> d = the pupillary diameter
> λ = the wavelength of the light that constitutes the point object

When two point sources are viewed by an eye with a small pupil, two diffraction patterns are formed on the retina (Fig. 11-5B). If the diffraction patterns are too close together, the two points will not be resolved—the patient will see only one point. The minimum separation required for the points to be resolved occurs when the peak of one of the Airy's disks falls on the center of the dark ring of the other disk. This minimum separation is the radius of the Airy disk.

Let us look at an example. *In order for two points of 555 nm to be resolved by a person with a 5.00 mm-diameter pupil, what is the minimum distance that must separate the peaks of the Airy disks?* After converting to meters, we have

$$\theta = 1.22\lambda/d$$
$$\theta = 1.22(5.55 \times 10^{-7} \text{ m})/5 \times 10^{-3} \text{ m}$$
$$\theta = 1.354 \times 10^{-4} \text{ radians}$$

Converting to minutes of arc, we have

$$(1.354 \times 10^{-4} \text{ radians})(180°/\pi \text{ radians}) (60'/1°) = 0.47'$$

For a 5.00 mm diameter pupil, the peaks of the Airy's disks must be separated by at least 0.47'. If we repeat this calculation for a 2.00 mm diameter pupil, we find that the Airy's disks must be separated by at least 1.16'. As the pupil becomes smaller, the diffraction patterns becomes larger; consequently the patterns (and point sources) must be further from each other in order to be resolved (Fig. 11-5C).[1]

---

[1] The packing density of the retinal photoreceptors limits our ability to resolve detail less than about 0.50' arc. In the case of a 5.00 mm diameter pupil, resolution is not likely to be limited by diffraction but by the density of the photoreceptors. As the pupil diameter decreases to about 2.00 to 3.00 mm, diffraction becomes the limiting factor.

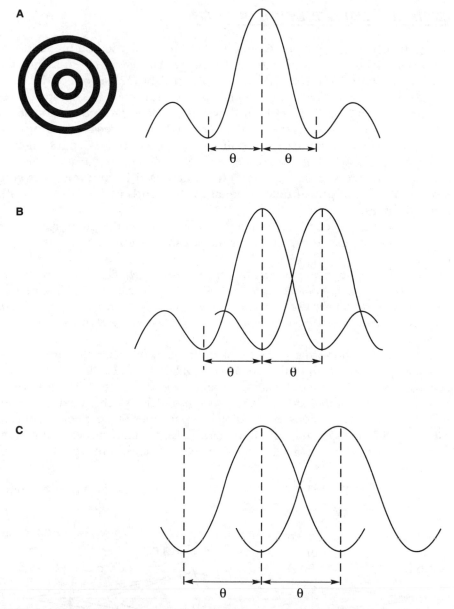

FIGURE 11-5A. The diagram on the left shows the diffraction pattern of light formed on the retina in viewing through an aperture with a small diameter. In the diagram on the right, which is a profile of the light distribution in the diffraction pattern, the peaks represent bright areas and troughs represent dark areas. The peak and first trough (dark ring) are referred to as *Airy's disk*. The radius of Airy's disk is designated as θ. **B.** Two objects cannot be resolved unless the peaks of the two Airy's disks are separated by at least the radius of Airy's disk (i.e., the peak of one disk falls on the trough of the other disk). In this diagram, the peak of one disk falls on the trough of the other disk; therefore resolution is not limited by diffraction. **C.** As the pupil becomes smaller, the diameter of the Airy disk increases. Consequently the point sources must be separated by a greater distance in order to be resolved (i.e., for the observer to see two point sources rather than one).

DEPTH OF FIELD AND DEPTH OF FOCUS

An object such as the optotype **E** does not have to be focused on the retina for us to resolve its details. As long as the retinal blur circles are not too large, the optotype can be resolved. In Figure 11-6, the patient (an uncorrected 3.00 D refractive myope who is an absolute presbyope) can resolve the optotype over the distance from X to Z. This distance, which can be expressed in diopters or linear units, is referred to as the *depth of field*. **When expressed in diopters, the depth of field is centered on point Y.** Conjugate to the depth of field is the *depth of focus*, which is the distance from X′ to Z′. This distance can also be expressed in diopters or linear units. **When expressed in diopters, it is centered on Y′. The depth of field is equal to the depth of focus when both are in diopters.**

The extent of the depth of field depends primarily on the pupil diameter. A small pupil decreases the size of the blur circles and thereby increases the depth of field.

Let us look at an example. *An absolute presbyope wears a near correction of +2.50 D. His total depth of focus is 0.50 D. What is his linear range of near vision when he wears his presbyopic correction? What would be his linear range of clear vision if he wore a near correction of +1.00 D? (Assume that the patient is emmetropic.)*

Figure 11-7A shows the patient looking through the +2.50 D correction. A point that is 40.00 cm from the eye is conjugate with the retina. What is the patient's depth of field? Recall that the depth of field (in diopters) is equal to the depth of focus (in diopters). This 0.50 D depth of field is centered at the dioptric distance of 2.50 D. Therefore the dioptric boundaries of clear near vision are 2.50 +/− 0.25 D, or 2.75 and 2.25 D. In linear units, the patient sees clearly from 36.36 to 44.44 cm when looking through the +2.50 D lens. Although this patient

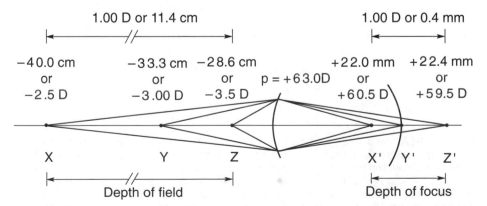

FIGURE 11-6. The depth of field is conjugate to the depth of focus. Although the depth of field and depth of focus are dioptrically equal (1.00 D), they are not linearly equal (11.4 cm versus 0.4 mm). (The 3.00 D myopic eye in this figure is uncorrected and unable to accommodate.)

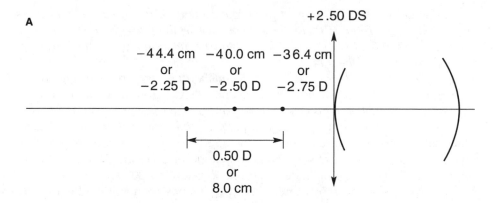

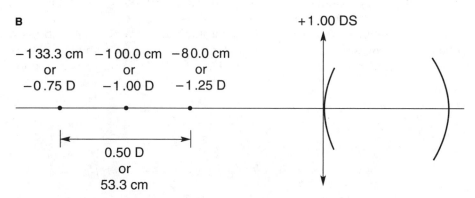

FIGURE 11-7. Depth of field for an absolute presbyope, whose total depth of field (and focus) is 0.50 D, when looking through **(A)** a +2.50 DS near correction and **(B)** a +1.00 DS near correction. (Assume that the patient is an emmetrope.) Although the depth of field is dioptrically the same at both distances (0.50 D), it is not linearly the same (8.0 versus 53.3 cm).

is an absolute presbyope, he is still able to see objects over a range of about 8.08 cm due to his depth of field.

Now, let us determine this absolute presbyope's range of clear vision when wearing a +1.00 D lens. As indicated in Figure 11-7B, a point at 100.00 cm anterior to the cornea is conjugate with the retina. The depth of field is centered dioptrically at 1.00 D: its dioptric boundaries are 1.25 and 0.75 D. These correspond to linear boundaries of 80.00 and 133.33 cm, for a range of 53.33 cm. It is important to note that although the dioptric depth of field (and dioptric depth of focus) does not change as the distance changes, the linear depth of field depends on the distance: at 40.00 cm it is 8.08 cm, and at 100 cm it is 53.33 cm.

Let us do another problem. *A presbyope looking through her bifocal add is able to see clearly from 25.00 to 100.00 cm. Her depth of field is +/−0.50 D (i.e., the total depth of field is 1.00 D). What is her true amplitude of accommodation? What is the power of the add?*

By *true (or actual) amplitude of accommodation,* we are referring to the change in the eye's dioptric power that is due solely to accommodation and *not* due to depth of field. In this case, the patients, range of clear vision, expressed in diopters, is from 4.00 to 1.00 D. The *apparent amplitude of accommodation,* which takes into account the depth of field, is 3.00 D (i.e., 4.00 D − 1.00 D = 3.00 D). Since 1.00 D of this apparent amplitude of accommodation is due to depth of field, the *true* amplitude of accommodation is 2.00 D.

For a presbyope to resolve near objects, plus power must be added to the distance prescription. As we learned in Chapter 8, the plus power that is added to the distance correction is called an *add* (Fig. 11-8). Through the add, the nearest clear distance is 25.00 cm in linear units or 4.00 D in dioptric units. Of this 4.00 D, 2.00 D is due to accommodation and 0.50 D to the depth of focus. The add provides the remaining power. Hence, the add has a power of 4.00 D − 2.00 D − 0.50 D = 1.50 D (Fig. 11-9A).

There is another approach to determine the add power. Without the add, distant objects are seen clearly. When looking through the add, the farthest distance that can be seen clearly is 100 cm (Fig. 11-9B). The add focuses the eye

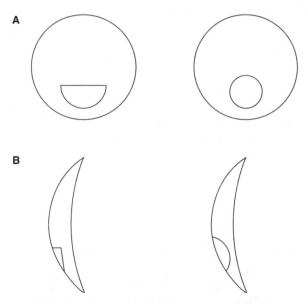

FIGURE 11-8A. Flattop and round bifocal adds. Not shown is a variable-focus lens, sometimes called a no-line bifocal. In such a lens, the plus power gradually increases going from the center of the lens toward its bottom. **B.** Cross sections of a bifocal lens. The adds in these bifocals have a higher index of refraction than the distance lenses.

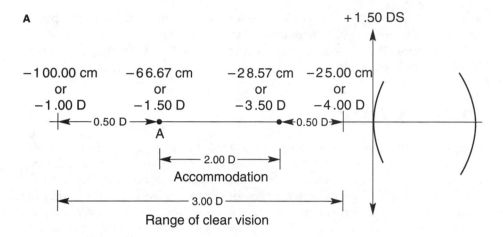

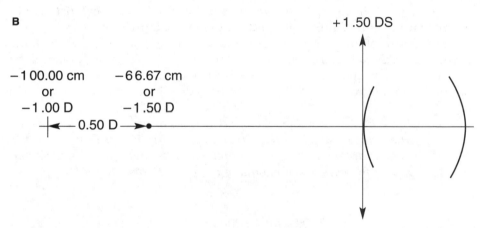

FIGURE 11-9. A presbyope, fully corrected for distance and viewing through her add, has a range of clear vision that extends from 25.00 (or 4.00 D) to 100.00 cm (1.00 D). If the patient did not have a +/–0.50 D depth of field, her range of clear vision would be from A (–1.50 D or –66.7 cm) to B (–3.50 D or –28.57 cm); therefore the true amplitude of accommodation (as measured at the spectacle plane) is 2.00 D. Since the patient's NPA is 25.00 cm, she must be wearing a +1.50 add (i.e., 0.50 D + 2.00 D + 1.50 D = 4.00 D). **B.** Since the farthest distance the patient can see is 100.0 cm and the depth of focus is +/–0.50 D, the patient must be wearing a +1.50 DS add. See text for details.

at a distance closer than 100 cm, but because of the depth of focus, the patient can see out to 100.00 cm. The depth of focus is +/− 0.50 D. If the add is + 1.50 D, the farthest distance that can be clearly seen is 1.00 D in dioptric units or 100.00 cm in linear units.

HYPERFOCAL DISTANCE

Consider a young emmetropic eye with a depth of focus of +/−0.50 D. The eye fixates a target located at infinity. As the target is slowly moved toward the eye, accommodation occurs. Assuming that accommodation is perfectly accurate, the eye remains focused on the object. The depth of focus is centered on the eye's fixation point and extends both toward and away from the eye. Eventually the eye will be focused at a distance—the *hyperfocal distance*—where the farthest extent of the depth of field is infinity. When the eye is focused at the hyperfocal distance, infinitely distant objects are seen clearly because they are within the depth of field. From Figure 11-10, **we can see that the hyperfocal distance in dioptric units is half the total depth of field (in dioptric units).**

In the case of an emmetropic eye with a depth of focus of +/−0.50 D, the hyperfocal distance is 200.00 cm (or 0.50 D). When focused at this distance, the depth of focus extends from 0.50 D +/− 0.50 D, or 0.00 D to 1.00 D. This corresponds to a linear range of clear vision extending from infinity to 100.00 cm (Fig. 11-10).

Let us consider an example. *When taking pilocarpine,[2] a myopic patient's uncorrected distance visual acuity is 20/20 and her depth of field is +/−1.00 D. When the patient discontinues the pilocarpine and her pupil returns to its normal size, what is the maximum amount of myopia we expect to find?[3]*

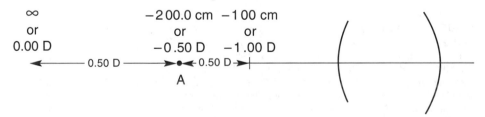

FIGURE 11-10. The hyperfocal distance (in diopters) is one-half of the total depth of field (in diopters). The eye is focused on A, which is at a distance of −0.50 D (200.00 cm). Since the depth of field is +/−0.50 D (i.e., the total depth of field is 1.00 D) and centered on A, objects at infinity can be resolved.

[2] Pilocarpine is a miotic (i.e., it decreases the diameter of the pupil), thereby increasing the depth of field and focus. This medication can be used to treat glaucoma.

[3] Assume the patient's best corrected visual acuity is 20/20 (i.e., when the patient's ametropia is fully corrected, the visual acuity is 20/20.)

We are asked to determine the maximum amount of uncorrected myopia that is consistent with a distance visual acuity of 20/20 and a hyperfocal distance of 100.00 cm. From Figure 11-11, we see that when an eye is focused at 100.00 cm (1.00 D), the depth of field extends to infinity, making 20/20 vision possible. Hence, the patient can have up to 1.00 D of myopia and still have uncorrected distance visual acuity of 20/20. (If the patient discontinues pilocarpine and the pupil returns to its normal size, the depth of focus will be less than +/−1.00 D and the distance uncorrected acuity will therefore be less than 20/20.)

A patient has a hyperfocal distance of 200 cm. What is the depth of field in linear units when the patient accommodates 2.50 D to view an object located 40.00 cm anterior to the cornea?

The hyperfocal distance, in diopters, is half the total depth of field. Since the patient's hyperfocal distance is 200.00 cm in linear units or 0.50 D in dioptric units, the depth of field in dioptric units is +/−0.50 D (i.e., the total depth of field is 1.00 D) (Fig. 11-12A). When focused on an object at 40.00 cm, the depth of field is centered at 2.50 D. Hence the depth of field extends from 2.00 to 3.00 D, or from 50.00 to 33.33 cm (Fig.11-12B).

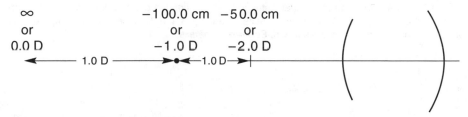

FIGURE 11-11. When taking pilocarpine, this patient can have up to 1.00 D of uncorrected myopia and still have 20/20 acuity. See text for details.

A

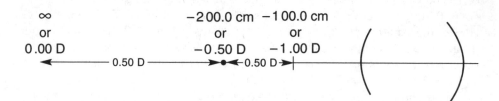

B

$$-50.00 \text{ cm} \quad -40.00 \text{ cm} \quad -33.3 \text{ cm}$$
$$\text{or} \quad \text{or} \quad \text{or}$$
$$-2.00 \text{ D} \quad -2.50 \text{ D} \quad -3.00 \text{ D}$$

|←——— 0.50 D ——→•←0.50 D→|

FIGURE 11-12A. Since the hyperfocal distance is 200.00 cm, the depth of field is +/–0.50 D (the total depth of field is 1.00 D). **B.** When fixating on an object at a distance of 40.00 cm, the range of clear vision is from 50.00 to 33.33 cm. See text for details.

P Self-Assessment Problems[4]

1. A 3.00 D myope who is fully corrected with contact lenses has a hyperfocal distance of 200.00 cm. His near point of accommodation is 10.00 cm. What is his true amplitude of accommodation?

2. A fully corrected 2.00 D hyperope has a total depth of field of 1.00 D. Through her spectacle add, her range of clear vision is from 100.00 to 25.00 cm. What is her range of clear vision through the distance portion of the spectacles?

3. Without any correction, a 1.00 D myopic presbyope has a near point of 20.00 cm. His total depth of field is 1.50 D. What is the furthest distance that this uncorrected myope can see clearly?

4. A presbyope wears bifocal spectacle lenses. Through the add, she can see clearly from 50.00 to 20.00 cm. Her total depth of field is 0.50 D. Assuming that she is fully corrected for distance, what is the power of the add?

5. A presbyopic myope wears bifocal spectacles that fully correct his 4.00 D of myopia. His total depth of field is 0.75 D. Through his bifocal add, he has a range of clear vision from 40.00 to 20.00 cm. What is his true amplitude of accommodation? Without his spectacles, what would be his near point of accommodation?

6. Without exerting any accommodation, an uncorrected 3.00 D myope can see clearly from 50.00 to 25.00 cm. The patient's true amplitude of accommodation is 2.00 D. When fully corrected for distance, what is the range of clear vision when the patient looks through a 2.00 D add?

---

[4] In solving these problems, assume that all measurements are made with respect to the spectacle plane.

Magnifying Devices 12

Because of disease, developmental abnormalities, or trauma, certain patients do not obtain satisfactory vision even though their ametropia has been fully corrected. These patients are said to have *low vision*. A patient with age-related macular degeneration, for instance, may have best corrected acuity[1] of 20/50. This patient will have difficulty reading the newspaper, correspondence from relatives and friends, and road signs while driving. As the population ages, the prevalence of low vision will increase. To obtain satisfactory vision, these patients may use magnifying devices such as a magnifying glass or a telescope. In this chapter we introduce these important clinical tools. This chapter is not intended to be a comprehensive discussion of low-vision devices.

MAGNIFICATION BY PLUS LENSES

A patient with low vision may require a magnifying device to resolve the print in certain reading materials, such as newspapers or correspondence. The most commonly prescribed near magnification device is a plus lens. The lens can be mounted in a hand-held magnifier, spectacles, a loupe positioned in front of the patient's spectacles, or a stand magnifier.

Lateral Magnification

Up to now, the magnification that we have discussed is lateral magnification.[2] As illustrated in Figure 12-1, lateral magnification is the ratio of the height (or other specified dimension) of the image to the height of the object. The orientation of the image (erect or inverted) is given by the sign of the lateral magnification. As we have previously discussed, the lateral magnification for a spherical refracting surface or lens is given by the ratio of the object vergence to image vergence:

---

[1] *Best corrected acuity* refers to the visual acuity obtained when the patient's ametropia is fully corrected.

[2] Lateral magnification is sometimes referred to as *transverse* or *linear magnification.*

159

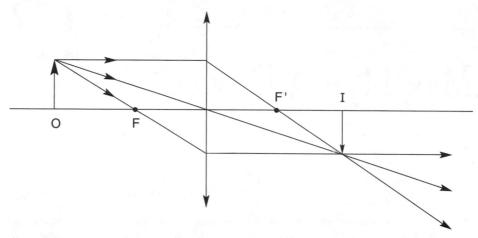

FIGURE 12-1. Lateral magnification is the ratio of the height of the image to the height of the object. In this case, the image is smaller than the object—the image is minified.

$$M_L = L/L'$$

In the special case of a lens that is surrounded by only one medium, such as air, lateral magnification is also given by the ratio of the image distance to object distance:

$$M_L = l'/l$$

When an object is located at the primary focal point of a plus lens, the image is formed at infinity (Fig. 12-2A). Specification of the lateral magnification is not useful in this situation. Effective magnification and lens angular magnification, our next topics, are sometimes used when the image is located at infinity.

Effective Magnification

Manufacturers of plus-lens magnifiers may specify magnification relative to a *reference distance* (sometimes called *standard distance*) of 25.0 cm. If the object is at the primary focal point of the plus lens, the image is located at infinity. The angle that this infinitely distant image subtends at the eye is compared to the angle the object subtends at the unaided eye when it (the object) is at 25.0 cm.[3] This magnification is sometimes referred to as *effective magnification*[4] or M_{25}.

Let us derive the formula for effective magnification. Figure 12-2A shows the formation of an image at infinity for an object located at the focal point of a plus

---

[3] We define an unaided eye as one that is not looking through a magnifier. [The eye is still considered unaided if it has ametropia and this ametropia is corrected with a spectacle lens (or contact lens)].

[4] Effective magnification is also called conventional or relative magnification.

A

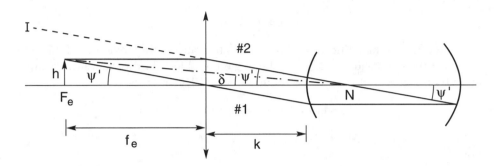

B

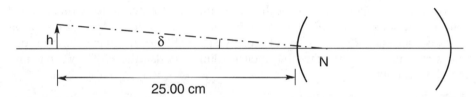

FIGURE 12-2A. When an object is placed at the focal point of a plus lens, a virtual image is formed at infinity. If the magnifying lens were not present, the nodal ray would follow the trajectory of the dotted-dashed line. **B.** Effective magnification is relative to a distance of 25.00 cm.

lens. Ray 1 passes undeviated through the optical center of the lens. After refraction, ray 2 passes undeviated through the reduced eye's nodal point.[5] We see that

$$\text{Tan } \psi' = h/f_e$$

where

> ψ' = the angle that the image subtends at the eye
> h = the height of the object
> f_e = the primary equivalent focal length of the lens

---

[5] Recall from Chapter 6 that a light ray directed at the nodal point is not deviated: the angle at which the ray intersects the nodal point is equal to the angle at which it emerges from the nodal point.

Now consider Figure 12-2B, where the object is located at the standard distance from the unaided eye, 25.0 cm. What angle does the object subtend at the eye? This is given by

$$\text{Tan } \delta = h/25.0 \text{ cm}$$

The effective magnification of the lens is the ratio of the angle that the image makes at the eye (with the lens) to the angle the object (at the standard distance of 25.0 cm) makes at the eye (without the lens). This ratio is

$$M_{25} = \tan \psi'/\tan \delta = (h/f_e)/(h/25.0 \text{ cm})$$

$$M_{25} = 25.0 \text{ cm}/f_e$$

but

$$f_e = 100.0 \text{ cm}/P_e$$

so

$$M_{25} = P_e/4$$

where

$$P_e = \text{the equivalent power of the lens}$$

For this formula to be correct, the object must be located at the primary focal point of the lens. Since effective magnification is measured relative to an arbitrary distance (i.e., 25 cm), it is not directly applicable to the many different distances at which patients may hold their reading material; therefore, M_{25} has limited clinical utility.

Angular Magnification of a Plus Lens

The *lens angular magnification*[6] (M_{ang}) is the ratio of the angle that the image produced by the magnifying lens subtends at the eye to the angle the object subtends at the unaided eye. Referring back to Figure 12-2A, the lens angular magnification is given by

$$M_{ang} = \frac{\tan \psi'}{\tan \delta} = \left(\frac{h/f_e}{h/(k + f_e)} \right)$$

$$M_{ang} = \frac{k + f_e}{f_e}$$

$$M_{ang} = P_e\left(k + \frac{1}{P_e}\right)$$

$$\boldsymbol{M_{ang} = kP_e + 1}$$

---

[6] Angular magnification is sometimes called *apparent* or *lens vertex magnification*.

where

$$k = \text{the distance from the lens to the cornea}$$

This formula assumes that the object is at the anterior focal point of the lens.

THE PROBLEM WITH MAGNIFICATION

As a plus lens is moved away from the eye (with the object remaining at the focal point of the lens), the angle subtended at the eye by the image (ψ') remains constant.[7] Simultaneously, the angle subtended by the object at the unaided eye (δ) decreases. Consequently, the lens's angular magnification increases. In fact, as the distance between the plus lens and the eye increases (with the object remaining at the focal point of the lens), it *appears* that the image is becoming larger. But this is an illusion caused by the shrinking of the field of view as seen through the lens; as the lens moves away from the eye, less of the image is seen through it. If you were to measure the retinal image size, however, you would find that it remains constant as the lens moves further from the eye (i.e., ψ' remains constant).

As long as the object is at the focal point of a plus lens, the retinal image is the same size regardless of the distance between the lens and the eye. This is clinically important because it is the size of the retinal image that determines if an object (e.g., newsprint) can be resolved.

When an object is held at the focal point of a plus lens, does the magnification produced by the lens change as the lens moves further from the eye? It depends on how you define magnification. The lens's angular magnification increases while the retinal image remains the same size. As you can well imagine, the various definitions of lens magnification have been a source of confusion for generations of clinicians. We can minimize this confusion if we do not think in terms of the magnification produced by a lens (Bailey, 1984). Examples illustrating this approach are given in the next section.

PRESCRIBING NEAR-PLUS MAGNIFIERS

Consider a 25-year-old patient who is having difficulty reading correspondence. The smallest print that this patient can read at 40.0 cm is 2 M.[8] Suppose the

---

[7] Figure 12-2 shows that $\psi' = h/f_e$. Therefore, for a given object with a height h located at the primary focal point of a given lens, ψ' remains constant.

[8] The size of print can be specified by its so-called *M size*. A 1 M optotype subtends an angle of 5 min of arc at the eye when it is 1m from the eye. The larger the print, the larger the M value. A 3 M optotype is three times as large as a 1 M optotype and 6 M print is twice as large as 3 M print, six times as large as 1 M print, one-third the size of 18 M print, and so on.

patient wishes to read print that is half as large—1 M print. What advice should we give to this patient?

The patient will be able to resolve the print that constitutes her correspondence as long as it subtends the same angle (at the eye's nodal point) as does 2 M print at 40.0 cm. One solution is for the patient to hold the 1 M print at a distance of 20.0 cm. When 1 M print is at a distance of 20.0 cm, it subtends the same angle as does 2 M print held at a distance of 40.00 cm.

Suppose that this patient's vision deteriorates so that in 2 years the smallest print that can be read at 40.0 cm is 5 M. If the patient wishes to read correspondence constituted of 1 M print, she could hold it five times closer to her eye—at a distance of 8.0 cm (Fig. 12-3A). This is probably not an acceptable solution because the patient is not likely to be comfortable holding reading material so close to the eye. Moreover, the accommodative demand is 12.5 D (i.e., 100 / 8.0 cm = 12.5 D); it is difficult to sustain this amount of accommodation for very long. What is an alternative?

What happens when the patient holds the reading material at the focal point of a lens that has a focal length of 8.0 cm (see Fig. 12-3B)? The parallel light rays that emerge from this +12.5 D lens (i.e., 100 / 8.0 cm = 12.5 D) subtend an angle at the eye (ψ') that is equal to the size of the print (1 M) divided by the equivalent focal length of the lens (8.0 cm). This is the same angle subtended by the 1 M print when it is held 8.0 cm from the (unaided) eye. Therefore, when the reading material is held at the focal point of a +12.5 D lens, the patient can read 1 M print. **Importantly, as long as the reading material is held at the focal point of the lens, the print will subtend the same angle at the eye (and the retina) regardless of the distance from the eye to the plus lens**. We have solved the patient's problem: she can hold 1 M print at a comfortable distance from her eyes and read it without accommodating if the print is situated at the focal point of a +12.5 D lens.

To repeat, the print subtends the same angle at the eye whether it is held 8.0 cm from the unaided eye or 8.0 cm from a +12.5 D lens (i.e., at the lens's primary focal point). The distance that the reading material must be held from the unaided eye in order to be resolved is defined as the *equivalent viewing distance*; the reciprocal of the equivalent viewing distance is the *equivalent viewing power* (Bailey, 1984). In the previous example, the equivalent viewing distance is 8.0 cm and the equivalent viewing power is +12.5 D.

Let us look at another example. *A fully corrected myopic patient with age-related macular degeneration can barely see 5 M print at a distance of 40.0 cm when looking through his bifocal add. If our goal is to allow the patient to read 2 M print, what power hand-held magnifying lens should we prescribe? How far should the lens be held from the reading material? How far should the lens be held from the patient's eye? Should the patient look through the magnifying lens with his distance correction or bifocal add?*

At first glance, this can appear to be a rather confusing problem. If we keep our wits and approach things one step at a time, it is not that complicated. The patient can read 5 M print when it is located at 40.0 cm. In order for the patient

A

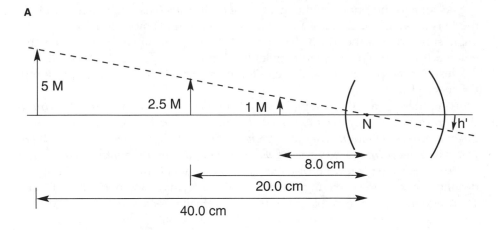

B

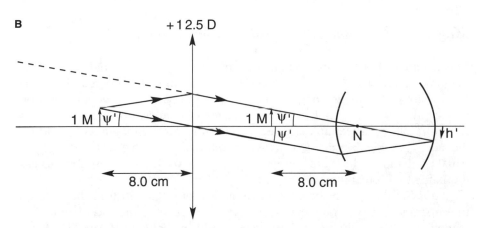

FIGURE 12-3A. Each of the following subtends the same angle at the eye's nodal point, resulting in the same retinal image size: 5 M print at 40.0 cm, 2.5 M print at 20.0 cm, and 1 M print at 8.0 cm. **B.** The equivalent viewing distance is 8.0 cm. 1 M print subtends the same angle at the eye whether it is located 8.0 cm from the unaided eye or at the focal point of a +12.5 D lens (whose focal length is 8.0 cm).

to read 2 M print, it must subtend the same angle at the eye as does the 5 M print at a distance of 40.0 cm. Since the 2 M print is 2.5*X* smaller than the 5 M print, it (the 2 M print) must be held 2.5*X* closer—at a distance of 16.0 cm—to subtend this angle (i.e., 40.0 cm /2.5 = 16.0 cm). Hence the equivalent viewing distance is 16.0 cm and the equivalent viewing power is +6.25 D. The patient could hold the reading material 16.0 cm from the eye and accommodate 6.25 D (i.e., 100 / 16.0 cm = 6.25 D). Alternatively, if the patient places the material at the focal point of a +6.25 D lens, no accommodation is required.

As long as the print is at the focal point of the plus lens, the patient can hold the lens at whatever distance from the eye that he finds most comfortable—the angle subtended at the eye is the same at all distances. Since the light rays that emerge from the plus lens are parallel to each other, they will be focused onto the retina if the patient looks through the plus lens with the distance portion of his spectacles.

Consider yet another example. *A patient has been able to read 6 M print at a reading distance of 40.0 cm when looking through her bifocal. She is now given a +10.00 D magnifying glass that she holds 10.0 cm from the page. What is the smallest print she can resolve when looking through the magnifying glass?*

The equivalent viewing distance is 10.0 cm. When material is held at this distance, it subtends an angle that is 4X larger than when held at 40 cm. Therefore the patient can read print that is 4X smaller—she can read 1.5 M print (i.e., 6 M / 4 = 1.5 M). Since the material is held at the focal point of the plus lens, the rays that emerge from this lens are parallel to each other; therefore the patient should look through the magnifier with her distance prescription.

Magnifying Lens and Bifocal Add in Combination

Will a patient obtain more magnification when looking through a hand-held magnifying lens with her distance prescription (keeping the object at the primary focal point of the magnifying lens) or with her bifocal add (keeping the object at the primary focal point of the add-magnifier combination)? As we will see from the following examples, it depends on how far the magnifier is held from the add. Consider a patient who wears bifocals that have a +2.50 D add. A +10.00 D hand-held magnifying lens (i.e., P_e = +10.00 D) is prescribed to assist the patient with reading.

Suppose the patient holds the magnifying lens 10.0 cm from her add (i.e., the separation between the magnifier and add is equal to the focal length of the magnifier). What is the equivalent power of this magnifier-add combination? To answer this question, we treat the magnifier-add combination as a thick lens. Using the thick lens formula from Chapter 6, we have

$$P_e = P_1 + P_2 - cP_1P_2$$

$$P_e = +2.50\ D + 10.00\ D - (0.1m/1.00)(+2.50\ D)(+10.00\ D)$$

$$P_e = +10.00\ D$$

When the magnifier is held one focal length from the add, the magnifier-add combination has the same equivalent power as the magnifier itself. Consequently, the size of the retinal image is the same whether the patient looks through the magnifier with her add or distance prescription.[9]

---

[9] Since the anterior principal plane of the magnifier-add combination is closer to the eye than the magnifying lens itself, the reading material should be held less than 10.0 cm from the magnifying lens if it is to be at the focal point of the magnifier-lens combination.

Now suppose the patient holds a magnifying lens less than 10.0 cm from her add, say at 5.0 cm from her add. What is the power of the system?

$$P_e = P_1 + P_2 - cP_1P_2$$

$$P_e = +2.50 \text{ D} + 10.00 \text{ D} - (0.05 \text{ m}/1.00)(+2.50 \text{ D})(+10.00 \text{ D})$$

$$P_e = +11.25 \text{ D}$$

When the distance between the magnifier and add is less than the focal length of the magnifier, the equivalent power of the magnifier-add combination is greater than that of the magnifier. Consequently, the size of the retinal image is larger when the patient looks through the magnifying lens with her add than when she looks through it with her distance prescription. This assumes that the reading material is held at the anterior focal point of the magnifier-add combination, which is less than 10.0 cm from the magnifying lens.[10]

Finally, what is the equivalent power when the magnifying lens is held further than 10.0 cm from the add, say at 15.0 cm?

$$P_e = P_1 + P_2 - cP_1P_2$$

$$P_e = +2.50 \text{ D} + 10.00 \text{ D} - (0.15 \text{ m}/1.00)(+2.50 \text{ D})(+10.00 \text{ D})$$

$$P_e = +8.75 \text{ D}$$

If the distance between the magnifier and add is greater than the focal length of the magnifier, the magnifier-add combination has less power than the magnifier. The patient is better off using her distance correction to look through the magnifying lens. This important finding is counterintuitive to both the clinician and the patient.

Let us summarize this section. How can a patient who wears bifocals maximize magnification when using a magnifying lens? She can do so if she looks through the magnifying lens with her add *while holding the magnifying lens closer to the add than its (the magnifying lens's) focal length.* However, if the magnifying lens is held further from the add than its focal length, the patient experiences less magnification; she is better off looking through the magnifier with the distance prescription. To ensure that the low-vision patient is obtaining the proper magnification, it is important to give instruction on the use of the magnifier and then for the patient to demonstrate to you that he or she can use the magnifier properly.

Fixed-Focus Stand Magnifiers

A plus lens can be mounted in a stand that rests on the reading material. Such a *stand magnifier* is illustrated in Figure 12-4. A fixed distance that is generally

---

[10] When the reading material is held at the anterior focal point of the magnifier-add combination, the light rays that emerge from this combination are parallel. They are incident on the distance prescription (which is behind the add) and focused onto the retina.

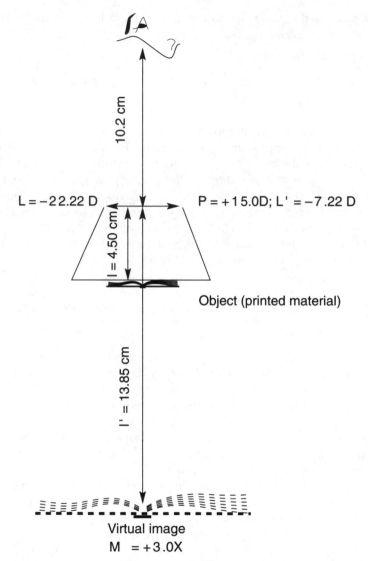

$$L = -2\,2.22\,D \qquad P = +1\,5.0D;\ L' = -7\,.22\,D$$

10.2 cm

l = 4.50 cm

Object (printed material)

l' = 13.85 cm

Virtual image

$$M = +3.0X$$

FIGURE 12-4. The distance from the plus lens of a stand magnifier to the reading material is less than the focal length, resulting in an enlarged virtual image. Here, the lateral magnification of the image is 3.0X. Since the equivalent viewing distance is 8 cm, the laterally magnified material can be up to 3.0X this distance from the eye—24.0 cm—and still be resolved. See text for further details.

shorter than the focal length of the lens separates the lens and the reading material. Consequently, an enlarged virtual image is formed.

Let us consider an example. *A patient can read 5M print when it is held 40.0 cm from his spectacles. You prescribe a stand magnifier that contains a lens with an equivalent power (P_e) of +15.00 D.*[11] *The lens is at a fixed distance of 4.50 cm from the reading material. How close must the patient's eye be to the plus lens for him to read 1 M print?*

For the patient to read 1 M print, it must subtend an angle that is 5.0X greater than it does at 40.00 cm. The equivalent viewing distance is 8.0 cm (40.0 cm / 5.0 = 8.0 cm), and the equivalent viewing power is +12.5 D. The patient could resolve 1 M print if it were held 8.0 cm from the unaided eye (assuming that he could accommodate 12.5 D) or if he held it at the focal point of a +12.5 D lens. Now, let us return to the stand magnifier.

Where is the image formed by the stand magnifier located, and how much is it magnified? Since the object is located within the focal length of the lens, a virtual image is formed. The image distance is

$$L' = L + P$$

$$L' = [(1.00)(100)/-4.50 \text{ cm}] + 15.00\text{D}$$

$$L' = -22.22 \text{ D} + 15.00 \text{ D}$$

$$L' = -7.22 \text{ D}$$

$$L' = 1/l'$$

$$-7.22\text{D} = (1.00)(100)/l'$$

$$l' = -13.85 \text{ cm}$$

This virtual image is located 13.85 cm from the lens (Fig. 12-4). The lateral magnification is

$$M_L = L/L'$$

$$M_L = -22.22 \text{ D}/-7.22 \text{ D}$$

$$M_L \sim +3.0X$$

We have already determined that the equivalent viewing distance is 8.00 cm. Since the image is enlarged (due to lateral magnification) by a factor of 3.0X, the reading material can be located 3.0X farther from the eye, at a distance of 24.00 cm. Since the image is located 13.85 cm from the plus lens of the stand magni-

---

[11] In this case, we are treating the stand magnifier lens as a thin lens. For clinical applications, it is important to know the equivalent power and image distance. Nowakowski (1994) explains how these values can be determined and provides tables that give these values for certain stand magnifiers. Also see Bailey (1981, 1983).

fier, the eye must be no further than 10.2 cm from the lens (24.00 cm − 13.85 cm ~ 10.2 cm) for 1 M print to be resolved.[12]

Closed-Circuit Television

Closed-circuit television (CCTV) is sometimes prescribed for the low-vision patient. With these devices it is possible to enlarge the reading material by zooming in on it, allowing the patient to remain at a comfortable distance from the television screen. Certain patients benefit from the device's capacity to reverse the contrast of the print (so that there is white print on a black background rather than black print on a white background).

Your patient can read 6 M print at a distance of 30.0 cm. She would like to read 1 M print when at a distance of 40.0 cm from the screen of a CCTV. By how much should the CCTV magnify the print?

The patient can read 1 M print if it is held at a distance of 5.0 cm from her eyes (30.0 cm / 6 = 5.0 cm). Therefore the equivalent viewing distance is 5.0 cm. If the patient wishes to read 1 M print when it is at a distance of 40.0 cm, the CCTV must magnify it by a factor of 8X to compensate for increasing the reading distance by a factor of 8.0X (40.0 cm / 5.0 cm = 8.0X).[13] [When 1 M print is magnified by a factor of 8.0X, it becomes 8 M print. Both 1 M print at 5.0 cm from the eye and 8 M print at 40.0 cm from the eye subtend the same angle (as does 6 M print at a distance of 30.0 cm).]

More on Near Magnification Devices

The goal of this discussion is to elaborate on the concept of magnification and to provide some examples of the application of this knowledge to simple clinical cases. There is much more to learn regarding the use of magnifying lenses in low-vision practice. At the conclusion of this chapter, suggested readings are given that discuss the clinical use of magnifying lenses in more detail.

TELESCOPES

A low-vision patient's distance vision can often be improved by using a telescope. Generally, a telescope is focused for infinity, but—as we will learn—telescopes can be adapted for near-vision use.

When an emmetrope or corrected ametrope uses a telescope to view an infinitely distant object, the light rays that enter the telescope have zero vergence,

---

[12] To see the image clearly, the patient must accommodate 4.17 D (i.e., 100 / 24.0 cm = 4.17 D) or look through a +4.17 D lens.

[13] Since the patient is 40.0 cm from the screen, she must accommodate 2.50 D or look through a +2.50 D lens.

as do the light rays that exit the telescope. Since the telescope does not have (finite) focal points, it is referred to as an *afocal* optical system.

Galilean Telescopes

The design of a *Galilean telescope*[14] is given in Figure 12-5A. For an infinitely distant object, a converging *objective* lens forms an image at the primary focal point of the *eyepiece*,[15] which is a negative lens. Since both the object and the image are at infinity (the bundle of rays entering the telescope are parallel and the rays emerging from the telescope are also parallel), lateral magnification is not appropriate; instead, the angular magnification is specified.

From Figure 12-5A, we see that

$$M_{ang} = tan\ \psi'/tan\ \psi = (h/f_2)/(h/f_1)$$

$$M_{ang} = f_1/f_2 = P_2/P_1$$

where

f_1 = the focal length of the objective
f_2 = the focal length of the eyepiece
P_1 = the power of the objective
P_2 = the power of the eyepiece

Note that the relative positions of the rays entering the objective are unchanged when they emerge from the eyepiece (i.e., ray 1 is on top and ray 4 is on bottom). Thus, the image is *erect*. Since the eyepiece is a negative lens, we must place a minus sign in front of the formula for magnification (a fudge factor) to obtain a positive value:

$$M_{ang} = -P_2/P_1$$

Or you may ignore the signs and just remember that a Galilean telescope creates an erect image.

Keplerian Telescopes

Unlike a Galilean telescope, both the objective and eyepiece of a *Keplerian telescope* are positive lenses. The objective images an infinitely distant object at the primary focal point of the eyepiece (Fig. 12-5B). We see that the angular magnification is

---

[14] Galilean telescopes are sometimes called *Dutch* telescopes.
[15] The eyepiece is also referred to as the *ocular lens*.

A   Galilean

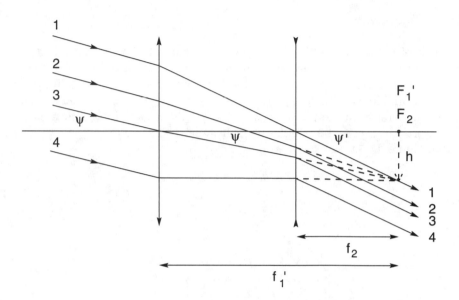

B   Keplerian

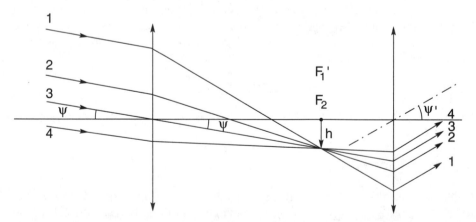

FIGURE 12-5A. A Galilean telescope, which consists of a weak positive objective lens and a stronger minus eyepiece, produces positive angular magnification. **B.** A Keplerian telescope, which consists of a weak positive objective and a stronger positive eyepiece, produces negative angular magnification, unless it is adapted with an inverting element (such as a prism). The *tube length* of a telescope is the distance between the objective and eyepiece.

$$M_{ang} = tan\ \psi'/tan\ \psi = (h/f_2)/(h/f_1)$$

$$M_{ang} = f_1/f_2 = P_2/P_1$$

where

f_1 = the focal length of the objective
f_2 = the focal length of the eyepiece
P_1 = the power of the objective
P_2 = the power of the eyepiece

In contrast to a Galilean telescope, the rays that emerge from the eyepiece of a Keplerian telescope are in the reverse order of the rays that enter the objective (i.e., entering the objective, ray 1 is on top, but it exits the eyepiece on bottom). Hence, the image is *inverted*. A minus sign is placed in front of the formula to indicate the proper orientation:

$$M_{ang} = - P_2/P_1$$

This is the same formula that we obtained for a Galilean telescope.

The Keplerian telescope in Figure 12-5B is referred to as an *astronomical telescope*. For clinical applications, it is necessary for a telescope to produce an erect image. With the use of prisms, an astronomical telescope can be converted into a *terrestrial telescope*, which produces an erect image. An advantage of Keplerian over Galilean telescopes is that they may provide the patient with a wider field of view: the patient sees a greater expanse of the visual world.

An Alternative Method of Determining a Telescope's Angular Magnification

The amount of light that enters an optical system is limited by the size of its *entrance pupil*. Light exits the system through its *exit pupil*. **For most telescopes, the entrance pupil is the objective lens. The exit pupil is the image of the objective lens as seen from the eyepiece side of the telescope**. The exit pupil of a telescope is also called a *Ramsden circle*.

For a Galilean telescope, the image of the objective lens (i.e., the exit pupil) is virtual and located within the telescope; for a Keplerian system, it is real and located outside of the telescope (Fig. 12-6). When the eyepiece end of the telescope is viewed from about 40 cm, the exit pupil for a Galilean system is seen as a small circle within the telescope, while the exit pupil for a Keplerian system is seen as a small circle floating in space.

The relative diameters of the entrance and exit pupils can be used to determine the magnification produced by a telescope. The formula is as follows:

M_{ang} = entrance pupil diameter/exit pupil diameter

A   Galilean

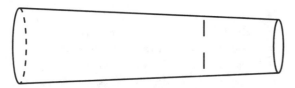

B   Keplerian

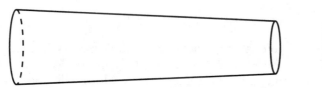

FIGURE 12-6. The exit pupil of a telescope is the image of the objective lens as seen from the eye-piece side of the telescope. **A.** For a Galilean telescope, the exit pupil can be seen floating within the tube; it is a virtual image. **B.** For a Keplerian telescope, the exit pupil can be seen floating in space, outside of the tube; it is a real image.

This formula is useful to the clinician because it provides a quick and straightforward method of determining (or confirming) the angular magnification produced by a telescope. Table 12-1 summarizes the characteristics of Galilean and Keplerian systems.

Lens Caps

Suppose that a telescope is used to view an object that is not at infinity but at, say, 100.00 cm from the telescope. This situation is illustrated in Figure 12-7, which shows a patient viewing an object with a Galilean telescope that has a +10.0 D objective and a −30.00 D eyepiece. Without the telescope, the object has a vergence of about −1.00 D at the eye; with the telescope, the vergence is −7.48 D. The telescope amplifies the object vergence, and this amplification makes it difficult (if not impossible) to use a telescope that is focused for infinity to view near objects.[16]

---

[16] When the telescope is focused for distance, the separation of the objective and eye-piece—the *tube length* of the telescope—is 6.67 cm.

TABLE 12-1. COMPARISON OF GALILEAN AND KEPLERIAN TELESCOPES

Characteristic	Galilean	Keplerian
Objective	Positive	Positive
Eyepiece	Negative	Positive
Image orientation	Erect	Inverted or erect[a]
Location of exit pupil	Within tube	Outside of tube

[a]Image-erecting systems (e.g., prisms) are included in Keplerian systems to create the terrestrial systems that are used for clinical purposes.

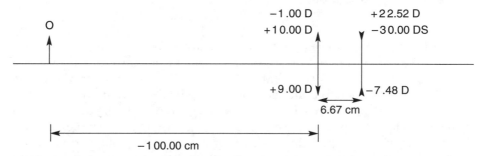

FIGURE 12-7. When a Galilean telescope (that is focused for distance) is used to view a near object, the vergence is amplified. Without the telescope the vergence would be about −1.00 D, but with the telescope it is −7.48 D. The separation of the objective and eyepiece—the *tube length* of the telescope—is 6.67 cm.

A telescope can be adapted for near use by placing a plus lens over the objective and positioning the object at the primary focal point of this lens. The plus lens images the object at infinity; therefore the rays that enter the telescope have zero vergence. A plus lens used is this manner is called a *lens cap*, and a telescope that is fitted with a lens cap is sometimes called a *telemicroscope* (Fig. 12-8).

Let us look at an example that we worked on earlier in the chapter. *A fully corrected myopic patient with age-related macular degeneration can barely see 5 M print at a distance of 40.0 cm when looking through his bifocal add. We wish to fit this patient with a +2.0X Galilean telescope. If our goal is to allow the patient to read 2 M print, what power lens cap should we prescribe? How far should the reading material be held from the telemicroscope?*

At the original distance of 40.0 cm, the patient can read 5 M print. To resolve 2 M print, the print must be held 2.5X closer to the eye (5M / 2M = 2.5), or at a distance of 16.0 cm (40.0 cm / 2.5 = 16.0 cm). This is the equivalent viewing distance. Since the telescope magnifies the print by a factor of 2.0X, the reading material can be twice as far from the telescope than the equivalent viewing distance—at a distance of 32.0 cm. For parallel rays to enter the telescope, the lens cap must have a focal length of 32.0 cm; therefore its power must be +3.13 D.

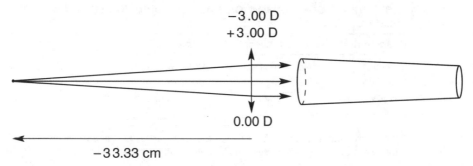

−3.00 D
+3.00 D

0.00 D

−33.33 cm

FIGURE 12-8. A lens cap is placed over the objective to create a telemicroscope. The working distance in this example is 33.33 cm.

Let us solve this problem by taking a slightly different approach. Since we would like the patient to be able to read 2 M print, the telemicroscope must provide magnification of 2.5*X* (i.e., 5 M/2 M = 2.5*X*). The telescope provides magnification of 2.0*X;* therefore the lens cap must provide magnification of 1.25*X* (i.e., 2.5 / 2.0 = 1.25). To do so, the reading material must be held 1.25*X* closer than the original distance—it must be held at a distance of 32.0 cm (i.e., 40.0 cm / 1.25 = 32.0 cm.) For the light rays to enter the telescope with zero vergence, the lens cap must have a focal length of 32.0 cm. Therefore, the lens cap must have a power of +3.13 D.

A spectacle-mounted device (either a plus magnifying lens or a telemicroscope) may be prescribed to enable a patient to see at near distances. Although the telemicroscope is more awkward than a magnifying lens and has a narrower field of view, it does offer an advantage. As we learned earlier in this chapter, if a magnifying lens is prescribed for the patient in the previous example, its power must be +6.25 D. To use this lens, the patient must place material at a distance of 16.00 cm from the lens. With the telesmicroscope, however, the patient places the material at a distance of 32.0 cm from the lens cap. This greater working distance may be preferable, especially if the patient intends to manipulate the viewed material.

BIBLIOGRAPHY

Bailey IL. Locating the image in stand magnifiers. *Optom Monthly.* 1981;72(6):22.
Bailey IL. The use of fixed focus stand magnifiers. *Optom Monthly.* 1981;72(8):37.
Bailey IL. Locating the image in stand magnifiers—An alternative method. *Optom Monthly.* 1983;74:487.
Bailey IL. Magnification of the problem of magnification of the... *Optician.* 1984;185:16.
Cole RG. Predicting the low vision reading add. *J Am Optom Assoc.* 1993;64:19.
Nowakowski RW. Primary Low Vision Care. Norwalk, CT:, Appleton & Lange; 1994.

P | Self-Assessment Problems

1. A Keplerian telescope consists of a +10.00 D objective and a +25.00 D eyepiece. (a) What is the angular magnification provided by the telescope? (b) What is the tube length of the telescope?

2. A 5.0X Galilean telescope consists of two lenses separated by a distance of 10.00 cm. What are the refractive powers of the objective and eyepiece?

3. When focused for infinity, the telescope in Problem 2 is used to view an object located 100.0 cm anterior to the objective lens. (a) How much accommodation is required to focus the object onto the retina? (b) What is the power of the lens cap that should be prescribed if your goal is for the patient not to accommodate (e.g., the patient is an absolute presbyope)?

4. When looking through a +2.50 bifocal add, a patient can read 6 M print at a distance of 40.0 cm. She desires to read 2 M print. (a) What is the dioptric power of the magnifier that will allow her to read 2 M print if the print is at the focal point of the magnifier and she views through the distance correction? (b) When viewing through the distance portion of her spectacles, at what distance should she be from the magnifier in order to obtain maximum magnification? (c) The patient occasionally must resolve print that is slightly smaller that 2 M. How can she obtain greater magnification with the magnifier that you prescribed in part (a) of this problem?

5. When looking through his bifocal add, your patient is able to read 5 M print at a distance of 40.0 cm. Using a magnifying glass that was given to him as a gift, he can read 1 M print if the print is held close to the focal point of the magnifying lens and he views through the distance portion on his spectacles. What is the dioptric power of the magnifying glass?

6. The patient in Problem 4 is not satisfied with the magnifying lens because she cannot hold it when using both hands to type on the keyboard of a computer. You decide to prescribe a telemicroscope. (a) If the telescope has an angular magnification of 2.0X, what is the dioptric power of the lens cap that you should prescribe? (b) How far should the cap be from the computer screen? (c) What is a limitation of the telemicroscope?

Retinal Image Size

13

The size of the image that falls upon the retina is influenced by the nature of the patient's refractive error and the manner in which it is corrected. The size of the retinal image is of clinical importance because clear and comfortable binocular vision requires that the retinal images of the two eyes be fused. When the retinal images of the two eyes are unequal in size, fusion becomes difficult and the patient may manifest asthenopic symptoms. This condition is referred to as *aniseikonia*.

LINEAR SIZE OF THE RETINAL IMAGE IN UNCORRECTED AMETROPIA

Figure 13-1 shows a reduced eye viewing an object that subtends the angle ω at the cornea. The axial length of the eye is given by a and the retinal image size is designated by x'. Assuming small angles, Snell's law gives us[1]

$$n\omega = n'\omega'$$
$$\omega' = \omega/n'$$

Also

$$\omega' = -x'/a$$

where the minus sign indicates that the image is inverted.
By substitution, we have

$$\omega/n' = -x'/a$$
$$x' = -\omega a/n'$$

but

$$A = n'/a$$

---

[1] For small angles, $\sin\omega \sim \omega$ (in radians).

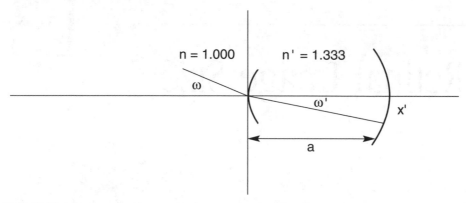

FIGURE 13-1. Linear retinal image size in uncorrected ametropia.

or

$$a = n'/A$$

so by substitution

$$x' = -\omega/A$$

From Chapter 7, we know that

$$A = F_{fp} + P_{eye}$$

where

F_{fp} = the far point vergence
P_{eye} = the power of the reduced eye

By substitution, we have

$$\boldsymbol{x'} = \frac{-\boldsymbol{\omega}}{\boldsymbol{F_{fp}} + \boldsymbol{P_{eye}}}$$

Table 13-1 shows the application of this relationship to the conditions of emmetropia, 5.00 D of uncorrected axial myopia, 5.00 D of uncorrected refractive myopia, 5.00 D of uncorrected axial hyperopia, and 5.00 D of uncorrected refractive hyperopia. Note that the (unfocused) retinal image in uncorrected refractive myopia and uncorrected refractive hyperopia is the same size as the image in the emmetropic eye. In comparison, the retinal image in uncorrected axial myopia is larger than in emmetropia, while the image in uncorrected axial hyperopia is smaller.

TABLE 13-1. LINEAR RETINAL IMAGE SIZE IN UNCORRECTED AMMETROPIA

Condition	F_{fp}	P_{eye}	Linear Size of Retinal Image
Emmetropia	0.00	+60.00	$-\omega/60$
Axial myopia	−5.00	+60.00	$-\omega/55$
Refractive myopia	−5.00	+65.00	$-\omega/60$
Axial hyperopia	+5.00	+60.00	$-\omega/65$
Refractive hyperopia	+5.00	+55.00	$-\omega/60$

In the following sections of this chapter, we examine the effect that correction of a refractive error has on the retinal image size. First, we determine the angular magnification produced by the spectacle lens itself, without consideration to the retinal image size. Next, we determine the angular magnification produced by the combination of the spectacle lens and the eye. Finally, the linear size of the retinal image in the corrected eye is examined.

SPECTACLE MAGNIFICATION

The lens used to correct a refractive error produces angular magnification. This magnification—referred to as *spectacle magnification*—is due to the lens itself, not the lens in combination with the power of the eye. Spectacle magnification is due to both the power of the lens (*power factor*) and the shape of the lens (*shape factor*).

Figure 13-2 shows parallel light rays incident on a plus lens used to correct a refractive error. The spectacle magnification due to lens *power* (i.e., the power factor) is by definition

$$M_{\theta(power)} = \theta'/\theta$$

but

$$\theta = -y'/f'_L$$

and

$$f'_L = 1/P_L$$

where

f'_L = the secondary equivalent focal length of the corrective lens
P_L = the equivalent power of the corrective lens

Therefore

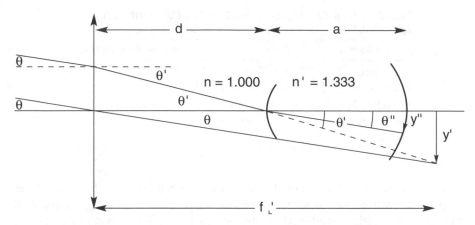

FIGURE 13-2. Magnification produced by a spectacle lens and eye in combination.

$$\theta = (-y')(P_L)$$

From the diagram, we also see that

$$\theta' = \frac{-y'}{f_L - d}$$

where d is the distance from the lens to the eye (i.e., the vertex distance). This relationship can be transformed to

$$\theta' = \frac{-y'P_L}{1 - dP_L}$$

By substitution and simplification, we have

$$M_{\theta(power)} = \frac{\theta'}{\theta} = \frac{1}{1 - dP_L}$$

This relationship gives the angular magnification due to the power of the correcting lens and is referred to as the *power factor.*

Considering only the power factor, how does the spectacle magnification produced by a −5.00 D lens compare with that produced by a +5.00 D lens? Assuming a vertex distance of 15.00 mm, we can use the above formula to determine that the angular magnification produced by a −5.00 D spectacle lens is .93X, while that produced by a +5.00 D lens is 1.08X. Taking into account only the power, a spectacle lens used to correct myopia produces angular minification, whereas a spectacle lens that corrects hyperopia produces angular magnification.

For a thin lens (which is a theoretical construct, since all lenses have some thickness), only the power factor is important. Ophthalmic lenses, however, have physical properties, including thickness, that affect the spectacle magnification. These physical properties contribute to the *shape factor*. The complete formula for spectacle magnification, showing both the power and shape factors, is as follows:

$$M_{(spectacle)} = [M_{(power)}] \times [M_{(shape)}]$$

$$M_{(spectacle)} = \left(\frac{1}{1 - dP_L}\right)\left(\frac{1}{1 - (t/n)\,P_v}\right)$$

In aniseikonia, the retinal images of the two eyes are unequal in size. This can be caused by *anisometropia*.[2] By manipulating the physical properties of a lens, including its thickness, we can influence the retinal image size. For instance, consider the following anisometropic prescription:

$$OD \quad -3.00 \text{ DS}$$
$$OS \quad -7.00 \text{ DS}$$

Within limits, the front vertex powers (P_v) and the thickness of the lenses can be adjusted to affect the angular magnification. By doing so, we can not only correct the refractive error but also make the two retinal image sizes more equal. Lenses used in such a fashion are sometimes referred to as *size lenses*.

ANGULAR MAGNIFICATION IN CORRECTED AMETROPIA

Let us derive the formula that gives the *angular* magnification in corrected ametropia. In the next section of this chapter, we use this formula to determine actual (physical) retinal image size. Returning to Figure 13-2, we see that the angular magnification produced by a spectacle lens *in combination with the eye* can be defined as θ'' / θ. From Snell's law, we also see that

$$n\theta' = n'\theta''$$

Since $n = 1$,

$$\theta' = n'\,\theta''$$

From the previous section, we know that

$$\frac{\theta'}{\theta} = \frac{1}{1 - dP_L}$$

---

[2] *Anisometropia* refers to the condition wherein the refractive error in one eye is substantially different from that in the fellow eye.

By substitution, we have

$$\frac{\theta''}{\theta} = \frac{1}{n'(1 - dP_{L})}$$

What does this formula tell us about the angular magnification in corrected ametropia? If the ametropia is corrected with spectacles (assume a vertex distance of 15.00 mm), the corrected myopic eye manifests angular minification relative to an emmetropic eye, while the corrected hyperopic eye shows angular magnification. When corrected with contact lenses, however, the vertex distance (d) is zero and the angular magnification is unaffected by the correction.

PHYSICAL IMAGE SIZE IN CORRECTED AMETROPIA

Although angular magnification is helpful in understanding image formation in corrected ametropia, we can also gain practical insights by determining the linear (physical) size of the retinal image. In Figure 13-2, we see that the linear image size is designated as y''. We also see that

$$\theta'' = -y''/a$$

or

$$\theta'' = -y''A/n'$$

Substituting in the formula from the previous section ("Angular Magnification in Corrected Ametropia"), we find

$$y''A = \frac{-\theta}{1 - dP_{L}}$$

But we know from Chapter 7 that

$$A = F_{fp} + P_{eye}$$

Therefore

$$y''(F_{fp} + P_{eye}) = \frac{-\theta}{(1 - dP_{L})}$$

In this formula, F_{fp} is the power of the lens in the *corneal plane* that corrects the refractive error. For now, we are interested in the condition where the eye is corrected with a spectacle lens. Recall from Chapter 7 that the power of the lens required to correct ametropia depends on the distance of the lens from the cornea (i.e., lens effectivity). Figure 13-3 illustrates a corrective lens at the corneal

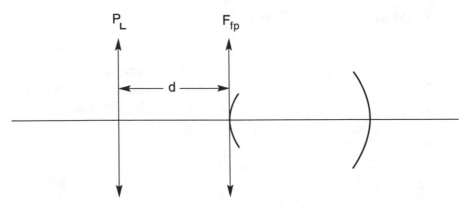

FIGURE 13-3. The lens power required to correct ametropia depends on the distance between the lens and the eye.

plane and a corrective lens located at the distance d from the cornea. From the figure, we can see that

$$F_{fp} = \frac{1}{f_L - d}$$

By substitution and rearrangement, we have

$$F_{fp} = \frac{P_L}{1 - dP_L}$$

By substitution and simplification, we obtain

$$y'' = \frac{-\theta}{P_L + P_{eye} - dP_L P_{eye}}$$

This formula gives us the linear size of the retinal image in the corrected ametropic eye. The relationship can be further simplified if the spectacle lens is placed at the anterior focal point of the eye, F_{eye}, as in Figure 13-4.[3] In this case,

$$d = f_{eye}$$

Since

$$f_{eye} = 1/P_{eye}$$

---

[3] The anterior focal point of the eye, like any focal point, is conjugate with infinity. If parallel rays emanate from the retina and strike the back of the cornea, they are focused at the anterior focal point, F_{eye}.

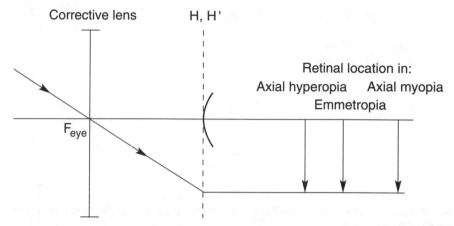

FIGURE 13-4. When a patient with axial ametropia is corrected with a spectacle lens placed at the anterior focal point of the eye, the size of the retinal image is the same as it is in emmetropia. The illustrated light ray passes undeviated through the optical center of the spectacle lens and anterior focal point of the eye, traveling horizontally once refracted by the eye. Since the ray contributes to the tip of the image, it can be used to determine the size of the retinal image.

then

$$d = 1/P_{eye}$$

Substituting in the above formula that gives retinal image size, we have

$$y'' = -\theta/P_{eye}$$

This formula allows us to calculate the size of the retinal image when the spectacle lens is at the anterior focal point of the eye.[4] For emmetropia and axial ametropia, the power of the reduced eye is +60.00 D. Consequently, when a patient with *axial* ametropia is corrected with a lens at the anterior focal point of the eye, the retinal image size is the same as in emmetropia, $-\theta/60$. This is referred to as *Knapp's law.*

A different effect is found in refractive ametropia. When a refractive myope is corrected with a lens at the anterior focal point of the eye, the retinal image size is minified to $-\theta/65$; for refractive hyperopia, the retinal image size is magnified to $-\theta/55$. These results are summarized in Table 13-2.

What is the retinal image size if we correct ametropia with contact lenses rather than spectacles? In this case *d* is equal to zero and we have

$$y'' = \frac{-\theta}{P_L + P_{eye}}$$

---

[4] The linear retinal image size in corrected ametropia can also be determined by multiplying the retinal image size in uncorrected ametropia by the spectacle magnification.

TABLE 13-2. LINEAR RETINAL IMAGE SIZE IN CORRECTED AMETROPIA

Condition	Linear Size of Retinal Image	
	Corrected with a Contact Lens[a]	Corrected with a Spectacle Lens[b]
Emmetropia	$-\theta / 60$	$-\theta / 60$
–5.00 D; axial	$-\theta / 55$	$-\theta / 60$
–5.00 D; refractive	$-\theta / 60$	$-\theta / 65$
+5.00 D; axial	$-\theta / 65$	$-\theta / 60$
+5.00 D; refractive	$-\theta / 60$	$-\theta / 55$

[a]When the refractive error is corrected with a contact lens, $\theta = \omega$.

[b]The spectacle lens is located at the anterior focal point of the eye.

Looking at Figure 13-3, we can see that when d is zero, P_L is equal to F_{fp}. Therefore we can rewrite the formula as:

$$y'' = \frac{-\theta}{F_{fp} + P_{eye}}$$

When the refractive error is corrected with a contact lens, θ is equal to ω (Figs. 13-1 and 13-2), making the formula the same as that used to calculate the size of the retinal image in uncorrected ametropia. Therefore, correcting an ametropic eye with a contact lens does not change the size of the retinal image from that in the uncorrected state (see Tables 13-1 and 13-2).

The differential diagnosis of axial ametropia from refractive ametropia is most often made by measuring the curvatures of the corneas. If both of the patient's corneas have the same radius of curvature, the ametropia is most likely axial in nature. If, however, the radii of curvature of the two eyes are substantially different, the ametropia has a refractive component. As we will discuss in the next chapter, it is relatively straightforward to measure the corneal radius of curvature clinically.

SUMMARY

Table 13-2 summarizes what we have learned about the size of the retinal image in corrected ametropia. An important clinical implication is that the nature of the correction (spectacle lens or contact lens) influences the retinal image's size. *Take the case of an anisometropic patient who has 1.50 D of myopia in one eye and 1.50 D of hyperopia in the fellow eye.[5] Should this patient wear spectacles or contact lenses?* The answer depends on whether the ametropia is axial or refrac-

---

[5] When one eye is myopic and the fellow eye is hyperopic, the condition is sometimes referred to as *antimetropia*.

tive. If it is axial,[6] the myopic eye has a larger retinal image, and the patient may manifest symptoms and signs of aniseikonia. Correction with spectacles results in comparable retinal image sizes (Knapp's law), whereas correction with contact lenses leaves the retinal images unequal in size.

If the ametropia is refractive rather than axial, the opposite holds true. In this case, the uncorrected retinal image sizes in the two eyes are the same, and correction with contact lenses would maintain this favorable situation. Correction with spectacles, however, would result in a larger retinal image size in the hyperopic eye, possibly resulting in aniseikonia. If the patient could not wear contact lenses and required spectacles, the shapes of the lenses (i.e., the shape factor) could be adjusted to minimize the difference in retinal image size.

---

[6] Axial ametropia can generally be distinguished from refractive ametropia based on keratometry readings (Chap. 14). If the corneal power is the same for the two eyes, the ametropia is axial.

P Self-Assessment Problems

1. A patient with the following spectacle prescription has LASIK performed on his right eye only.

$$OD -7.00 \text{ DS}$$
$$OS -5.00 \text{ DS}$$

The myopia is refractive, and prior to the laser procedure he was asymptomatic when corrected with either spectacles or contact lenses. Following the procedure, the right eye is plano. If your primary treatment goal is to avoid aniseikonia, should you prescribe spectacles (i.e., plano in the right eye and −5.00 DS in the left eye) or contact lenses (i.e., a contact lens for the left eye only)?

2. When refracted in the spectacle plane, we find that the following provides the best corrected distance acuity:

$$OD -6.00 \text{ DS}$$
$$OS -3.00 \text{ DS}$$

The patient's myopia is axial; you correct it with contact lenses. Compared to the right eye, how much larger (or smaller) is the left eye's image, expressed as a percentage?

3. A patient is fully corrected with the following spectacle prescription:

$$OD +7.00 \text{ DS}$$
$$OS +1.00 \text{ DS}$$

Compared to the angular magnification produced by the right lens, how much more (or less) is the angular magnification produced by the left lens? Express your answer as a percentage. (Ignore the shape of the lens.)

Reflection 14

Light rays that are incident upon a surface can be transmitted, absorbed, or reflected by the surface. In this chapter, we consider the reflection that is produced *by specular surfaces*—smooth (shiny) surfaces such as mirrors. **For a mirror, the angle that the reflected ray makes with the normal is equal to the angle that the incident ray makes with the normal** (Fig. 14-1). This is referred to as the *law of reflection*.

Not all surfaces are specular. *Nonspecular surfaces* are irregular and reflect incident light in various directions (Fig. 14-2). When light is incident on certain nonspecular surfaces, such as a blackboard, the light tends to be reflected evenly in all directions. A blackboard is an example of a *perfectly diffusing surface*.[1] When such a surface is viewed from different angles, it appears the same brightness—it does not appear shiny or glossy, as does a specular surface.

RAY TRACING: CONCAVE, CONVEX, AND PLANE MIRRORS

Concave Mirrors

Concave mirrors converge light; like converging lenses, they have plus power. Figure 14-3 shows parallel light rays incident on a converging mirror. After reflection, the rays intersect at the mirror's secondary focal point, F'.

Point C is the center of curvature of the mirror, and r is the radius of the sphere from which the mirror is formed. The radii are normal to the surface of the mirror. Note that with respect to the normal to the surface, the angle of incidence is equal to the angle of reflection. This is a basic property of mirrors.

As with lenses, ray tracing can be used to locate the image that is formed by a mirror. In Figure 14-4A, we see how four rays are used to locate an image. Ray 1 emerges from the object parallel to the optical axis and is reflected

---

[1] A perfectly diffusing surface is also referred to as a *cosine* or *Lambert surface*.

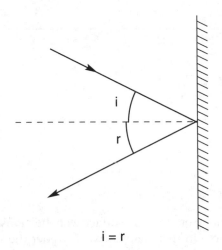

i = r

FIGURE 14-1. For a specular surface, the angle of reflection (*r*) equals the angle of incidence *(i)*. Both angles are specified with respect to the normal to the surface.

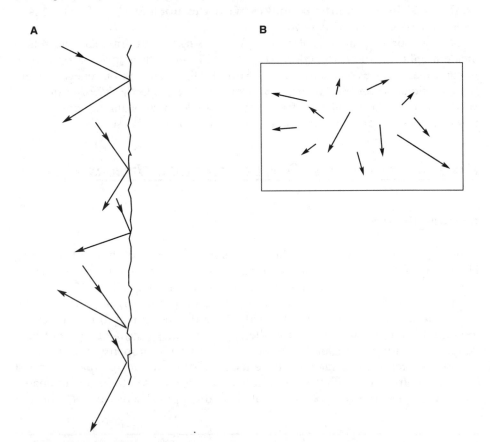

FIGURE 14-2. A nonspecular surface reflects light in various directions. **A.** Profile of a nonspecular surface. **B.** Direct face-on view of a nonspecular surface.

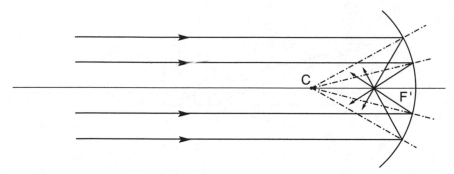

FIGURE 14-3. Parallel light rays, incident upon a converging mirror, are focused at the mirror's secondary focal point, *F'*. The dotted-dashed lines follow the radii that extend from the center of curvature (*C*) to the surface of the sphere. The radii are normal to the surface of the mirror.

through the secondary focal point.[2] Ray 2 strikes the mirror at the optical axis; the angles of incidence and reflection are symmetrical with regard to the optical axis. The third ray passes through the secondary focal point and is reflected parallel to the optical axis. Finally, ray 4 passes through the center of curvature, strikes the mirror perpendicular to its surface, and is reflected back through the center of curvature (i.e., since the angle of incidence is zero, the angle of reflection is also zero). The reflected rays intersect to form a real, inverted, and minified image.

A real image produced by a concave mirror is not always minified. As we can see from Figure 14-4B, when the object is situated between the center of curvature and the focal point, the inverted real image is larger than the object.

In the two examples we just discussed, the object is located further from the mirror than the focal point. What happens when the object is located within the focal length of the mirror? As is the case with a converging lens, an object located within the focal length results in an erect, virtual, and magnified image (Fig. 14-4C).

Convex Mirrors

A convex mirror diverges light; like a diverging lens, it has negative power. Figure 14-5A shows parallel light rays incident upon a convex mirror. After reflection, these rays appear to emerge from the mirror's secondary focal point, *F'*.

The same four rays that are used to locate the image formed by a concave mirror can be used to locate the image formed by a convex mirror. As can be seen in Figure 14-5B, a convex mirror forms a minified, erect, virtual image.

---

[2] As with a lens, the optical axis of a mirror connects the center of curvature and the focal point.

A

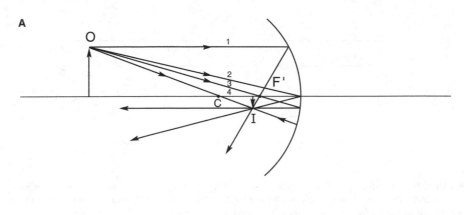

B

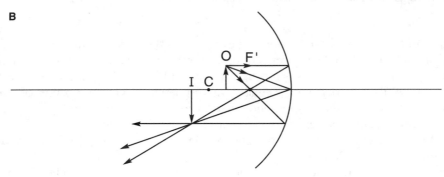

C

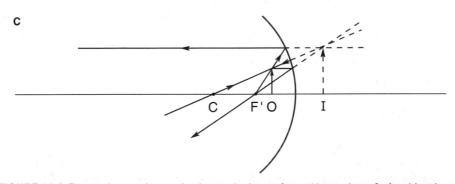

FIGURE 14-4. Ray tracing can be used to locate the image formed by a mirror. **A.** An object located outside of a converging mirror's focal length results in a real, inverted, and minified image. **B.** An object located between the focal point and center of curvature of a converging mirror results in a real, inverted, and magnified image. **C.** An object located within the converging mirror's focal length results in a virtual, erect, and magnified image.

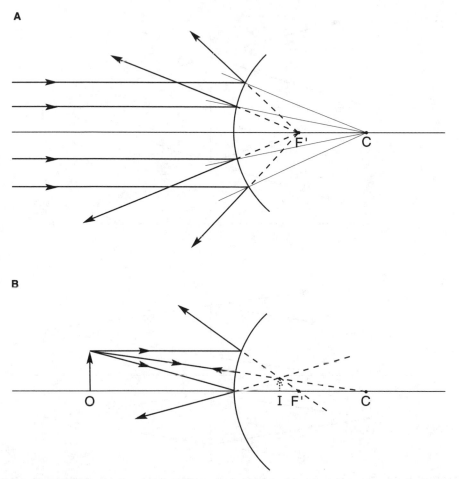

FIGURE 14-5A. Parallel rays, incident upon a convex mirror, appear to emerge from the secondary focal point, *F′*. The lines that extend from the center of curvature follow the radii and are perpendicular to the mirror's surface. **B.** Ray tracing shows that the image formed by this convex mirror is virtual, erect, and minified. The virtual image is located behind the mirror.

Plane Mirrors

A plane mirror has an infinite radius of curvature—it is flat. Unlike a concave or convex mirror, a plane mirror does not have power: it does not change the vergence of the light that is incident upon it.

Figure 14-6A shows an object that is located in front of a plane mirror. By applying the law of reflection to each of the light rays, we can locate the image. Note that the image is virtual and located the same distance from the mirror as is the object. Therefore if the object is 3.0 m in front of the mirror, the virtual image is 3.0 m behind the mirror.

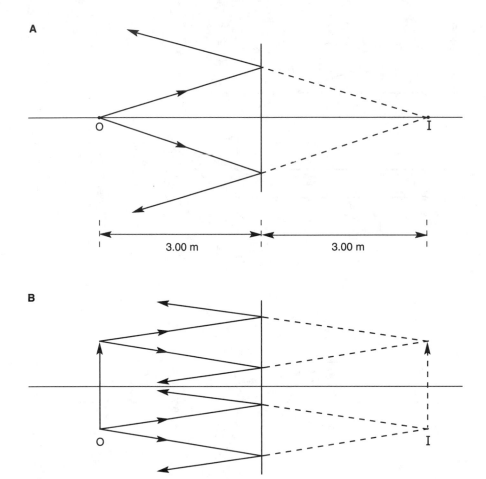

FIGURE 14-6A. The image formed by a plane mirror is virtual and located the same distance from the mirror as the object. **B.** The image formed by a plane mirror is the same size as the object.

What is the magnification produced by a plane mirror? In Figure 14-6B, the object is an arrow. As you can see, the separation of the top and bottom points of the arrow is equal to the separation of the images of these two points. The image produced by a plane mirror is the same size and orientation (i.e., erect) as the object—the magnification is a factor of one.

POWER OF MIRRORS

It is relatively straightforward to adapt the principles and formulae that apply to spherical surfaces to mirrors.[3] To do so, we must recognize that there is only

---

[3] Whereas the branch of optics dealing with refraction is referred to as *dioptrics*, the branch dealing with mirrors is *catoptrics*.

one medium (usually air), and that after reflection, the direction of the rays is reversed.

Recall from Chapter 2 that the power of a lens can be determined with the following relationship:

$$P = \frac{n' - n}{r}$$

Referring back to Figures 14-4 and 14-5B, we see that both the incident and reflected rays exist in the primary medium and that the direction of the rays is reversed after reflection. To use our linear sign convention, this reversal in direction must be indicated as follows:

$$n' = -n$$

Substituting, we have

$$P = \frac{-n - n}{2}$$

$$\boldsymbol{P = \frac{-2n}{r}}$$

If the mirror is in air ($n = 1$), then

$$\boldsymbol{P = -2/r}$$

As with a lens, the power of a mirror can be calculated directly from its focal length. Recall that the relationship between the power of a lens and the secondary focal length is

$$P = n'/f'$$

But for a mirror,

$$n' = -n$$

Thus, the relationship between the power of a mirror and the secondary focal length is

$$\boldsymbol{P = -n/f'}$$

If the mirror is in air, then

$$\boldsymbol{P = -1/f'}$$

Another useful relationship can be derived by equating the previous power formulae:

$$-2/r = -1/f'$$

or

$$\boldsymbol{r = 2f'}$$

This relationship tells us that the radius of curvature of a mirror is equal to twice its focal length.

Let us look at an example. *A concave mirror has a radius of curvature of 10.00 cm. Where is the focal point located with respect to the mirror's surface? What is the mirror's power?*

Our linear sign convention can be used to solve problems involving mirrors. Since the center of curvature of a concave mirror is to the left of the mirror, it is designated as a negative distance (Fig. 14-7). The focal length is calculated as follows:

$$r = 2f'$$
$$-10.00 \text{ cm} = 2f'$$
$$f' = -5.00 \text{ cm}$$

The focal point is located 5.00 cm to the left of the mirror's surface. The mirror's power is

$$P = -1/f'$$
$$P = -1/-.05 \text{ m}$$
$$P = +20.00 \text{ D}$$

THE VERGENCE (PARAXIAL) RELATIONSHIP

The vergence relationship can be used to locate the image produced by a mirror and to determine its magnification. However, we need to keep in mind that after reflection, the direction of the light is reversed.

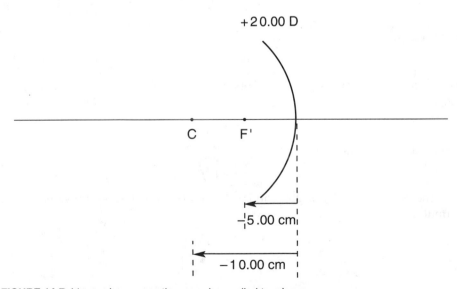

FIGURE 14-7. Linear sign conventions can be applied to mirrors.

Consider this example. *An object is located 80.00 cm in front of a concave mirror that has a radius of curvature of 33.33 cm. The object is 5.00 cm in height. Where is the image located? Is the image real or virtual? Is it erect or inverted? What is the height of the image?*

For a concave mirror, the center of curvature is located to the left the mirror's surface. This means that the radius of curvature is a negative distance (Fig. 14-8A). The power of this converging mirror is

$$P = -2/r$$
$$P = -2 / -.3333 \text{ m}$$
$$P = +6.00 \text{ D}$$

This makes sense, because we know that a concave mirror by definition has positive power.

The object vergence is

$$L = n/l$$
$$L = 1 / -0.80 \text{ m}$$
$$L = -1.25 \text{ D}$$

To determine the image vergence, we use the paraxial relationship

$$L' = L + P$$
$$L' = -1.25 \text{ D} + 6.00 \text{ D}$$
$$L' = +4.75 \text{ D}$$

Since the vergence is positive, the image is real and must be located to the *left* of the mirror. (Recall from Chap. 2 that a real image is formed by converging light rays and can be focused on a screen. Such an image can be formed only to the left of a concave mirror's surface.) Suppose we determine image distance with the same formula we use for lenses. In this case,

$$L' = 1/l'$$
$$l' = 1/ +4.75 \text{ D}$$
$$l' = +0.2105 \text{ m or } +21.05 \text{ cm}$$

This is not correct! The plus sign tells us that the image is located to the right of the mirror—but we know this is not the case (Fig. 14-8A). To properly convert the image vergence into the image distance, we must take into account the reversal in the direction of light that occurs after reflection. Therefore, for mirrors,

$$\boldsymbol{L' = -1/l'}$$

Returning to the sample problem, the image distance is properly calculated as follows:

$$l' = -1 / +4.75 \text{ D}$$

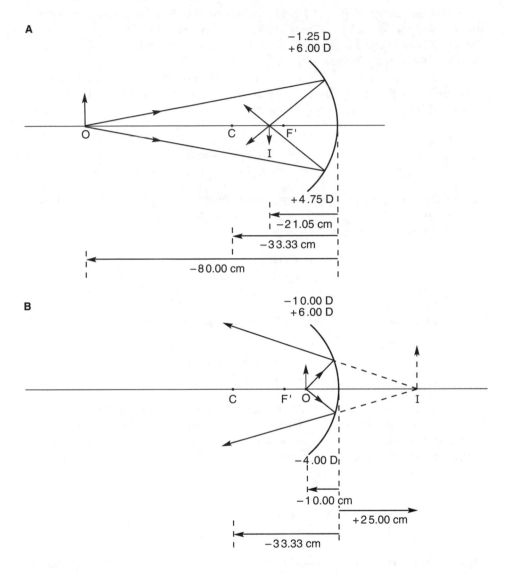

FIGURE 14-8. The paraxial relationship can be used to determine the location and size of the image formed by a mirror. For this and following diagrams in this chapter, the object vergence and mirror power are given at the top of the mirror and the image vergence is given below the mirror. See text for details.

$$l' = -21.05 \text{ cm}$$

The real image is formed 21.05 cm to the left of the mirror.

Now let us calculate the lateral magnification. From Chapter 3, recall that

$$M_L = L/L'$$

therefore

$$M_L = -1.25 / +4.75$$
$$M_L = -0.26X$$

This tells us that the image is minified and inverted. Its size is

$$(-0.26)(5.00 \text{ cm}) = -1.30 \text{ cm}$$

As with lenses, we can also calculate the magnification using linear distances. But because the light rays reverse direction after reflection, we must insert a minus sign into the equation:

$$\boldsymbol{M_L = -l'/l}$$

For our example, we have

$$M_L = -(-21.05 \text{ cm})/-(80.00 \text{ cm})$$
$$M_L = -0.26X$$

For this same mirror, locate the image if the object is located 10.0 cm in front of the mirror. Is the image real or virtual? Is it erect or inverted? What is the magnification?

The object vergence is

$$L = 1/l$$
$$L = 1 / -0.10 \text{ cm}$$
$$L = -10.00 \text{ D}$$

The image vergence is determined with the paraxial equation

$$L' = L + P$$
$$L' = -10.00 \text{ D} + 6.00 \text{ D}$$
$$L' = -4.00 \text{ D}$$

Since the vergence is negative, the image is virtual. It is formed by diverging rays and must exist 25.00 cm to the right of the mirror (Fig. 14-8B). We can confirm this by using the relationship for image vergence for mirrors:

$$L' = -1/l'$$
$$l' = -1 / -4.00 \text{ D}$$
$$l' = +0.25 \text{ m or } +25.00 \text{ cm}$$

What is the magnification? Using the vergence formula for lateral magnification, we have

$$M_L = L/L'$$
$$M_L = -10.00\ D/-4.00\ D$$
$$M_L = +2.50X$$

Hence the virtual image is erect and magnified.

Now consider an object located 20.00 cm in front of a convex mirror whose focal length is 25.00 cm. Where is the image located? Is the image real or virtual? Is it erect or inverted? What is the magnification?

Since the secondary focal point is located to the right of the mirror, it is designated with a positive sign (Fig. 14-9). The mirror's power is calculated as

$$P = -1/f'$$
$$P = -1/+0.25\ m$$
$$P = -4.00\ D$$

The object vergence is –5.00 D. Using the vergence relationship, we find

$$L' = L + P$$
$$L' = -5.00\ D + (-4.00\ D)$$
$$L' = -9.00\ D$$

Since the image vergence is negative, the image is virtual. Where is it located? From our understanding of mirrors, we know that a virtual image must be located to the right of the mirror. The distance is

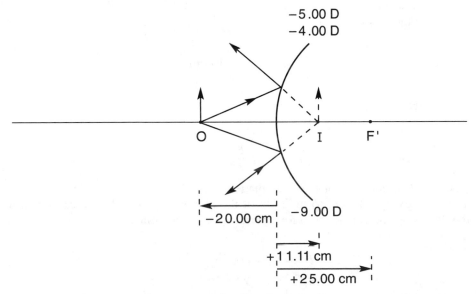

FIGURE 14-9. Another example of the use of the paraxial relationship to determine the location and size of the image formed by a mirror. See text for details.

$$L' = -1/l'$$
$$l' = -1/-9.00 \text{ D}$$
$$l' = +0.111\text{m or } +11.1 \text{ cm}$$

The magnification is given by

$$M_L = L/L'$$
$$M_L = -5.00 \text{ D}/-9.00 \text{ D}$$
$$M_L = +0.56X$$

The virtual image is erect and minified.

Before we move on, let us do one more problem. *An object 60.00 cm in height is located 200.00 cm from a plane mirror. Where is the image and what is its size?*

Recall that the virtual image formed by a plane mirror is the same size as the object and at a distance equal to the object distance. So for this example, the virtual image is located 200.00 cm behind the mirror and has a height of 60.00 cm. We can confirm this with the vergence relationship. Since the plane mirror has a power of zero, we have

$$L' = L + P$$
$$L' = (1/-2.00 \text{ m}) + 0$$
$$L' = -0.50 \text{ D}$$

Since the image vergence is negative, the image must be located to the right of the mirror. Its distance from the mirror is

$$L' = -1/l'$$
$$l' = -1/-0.50 \text{ D}$$
$$l' = +200.00 \text{ cm}$$

The magnification is

$$M_L = L/L'$$
$$M_L = -0.50 \text{ D}/-0.50 \text{ D}$$
$$M_L = +1.00X$$

These calculations confirm our conclusions from Figure 14-6: for a plane mirror, image distance is equal to object distance, and the image and object are the same height.

REFLECTIONS AND ANTIREFLECTIVE COATINGS

A transparent surface both transmits and reflects light. Take, for instance, a typical window. The window transmits light—you can see through it and someone on the other side of the window can see you. If you look closely, however, you can also see your reflection in the window—it acts as a mirror.

The amount of light reflected by a transparent surface is determined by the index of refraction of the primary medium (the medium in which the object is located) and the index of refraction of the secondary medium (the surface). As the difference in the indexes of the media increases, the amount of light that is reflected increases. For light rays that are perpendicular to a transparent surface, the fraction of light *(FR)* that is reflected is given by the following relationship:

$$FR = \left[\frac{n' - n}{n' + n} \right]^2$$

Light is reflected off the surfaces of ophthalmic lenses. Not only do these reflections reduce the amount of light that is transmitted by the lens but they may also be noticeable to people looking at the lenses (Fig. 14-10). From the above formula, we can see that lenses with higher refractive indices will reflect more light. A polycarbonate lens with an index of 1.586 reflects 5.13% of the light incident on its front surface, while 6.72% is reflected from a flint glass lens with an index of 1.700.

Bothersome reflections can be reduced by applying a thin, transparent *antireflective coating* to the surface of a lens. These coatings are effective because they cause destructive interference between the light that is reflected from the front surface of the coating and light reflected from the front surface of the lens (Fig. 14-11). For this to occur, the light reflected from the front surface

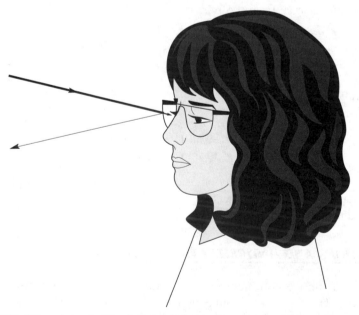

FIGURE 14-10. Although most of the light that is incident upon a lens is transmitted, a small fraction of the incident light is reflected by the surface.

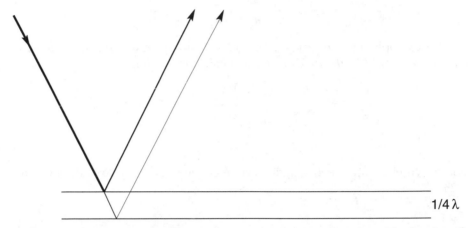

FIGURE 14-11. An antireflective coating, because of its thickness, causes destructive interference between the light rays that are reflected off the front surface of the coating and the front surface of the lens.

of the coating must be 180 degrees out of phase with the light that is reflected by the surface of the lens.

The coating is selected to be maximally effective for only one wavelength, typically in the yellow region of the spectrum. To obtain destructive interference, the light that is reflected from the front surface of the lens must travel one-half wavelength further than the light reflected by the front surface of the coating. Consequently, the coating must be an odd number of quarter wavelengths thick (i.e., one-quarter, three-quarters, etc., wavelengths thick). Because the destructive interference reduces reflections in primarily the yellow region of the spectrum, the remaining reflections from the lens may appear slightly purple.[4]

To obtain maximal destructive interference, the amount of light reflected from the two surfaces should be equal (Fig. 14-11). This occurs when the following condition is met:

FR off the surface of the coating = *FR* off the surface of the lens

$$\left(\frac{1 - n_c}{1 + n_c} \right)^2 = \left(\frac{n_c - n_g}{n_c + n_g} \right)^2$$

where

n_g = the refractive index of the lens
n_c = the refractive index of the coating

This relationship can be simplified to

---

[4] The purple color is due to an additive mixture of short- and long-wavelength light that is reflected off the lens.

$$n_c = \sqrt{n_g}$$

Let us apply this formula. *A crown glass lens requires an antireflection coating. What should be the index of refraction of the coating?*

$$n_c = \sqrt{n_g}$$
$$n_c = \sqrt{1.52}$$
$$n_c = 1.23$$

For crown glass, an effective antireflection coating[5] has an index of refraction of 1.23.

PURKINJE IMAGES

The four primary refracting surfaces of the eye—the anterior surface of the cornea, the posterior surface of the cornea, the anterior surface of the lens, and the posterior surface of the lens—all act as mirrors and reflect light. If you shine a penlight onto a patient's eye, you see a bright reflection off the anterior surface of the cornea. The refection is bright because of the relatively large difference between the indexes of air and the cornea (n = 1.376). Under optimal viewing conditions, it is also possible to see considerably dimmer reflections from the other three ocular surfaces. These four reflected images are called *Purkinje (or Purkinje-Sanson) images.*

Table 14-1 lists the four Purkinje images and their characteristics, and Figure 14-12 shows their approximate locations. Since the first three images are formed by convex reflecting surfaces, they are virtual and erect. Purkinje image IV, because it is formed by the posterior surface of the lens, which is concave, is real and inverted.

TABLE 14-1. SUMMARY OF CHARACTERISTICS OF PURKINJE IMAGES

Number	Source	Location[a]	Nature	Brightness[b]
I	Anterior cornea	3.85 mm	Virtual, erect	1
II	Posterior cornea	3.77 mm	Virtual, erect	2
III	Anterior lens	10.50 mm	Virtual, erect	3
IV	Posterior lens	3.96 mm	Real, inverted	3

[a]Location with respect to the corneal apex.
[b]Comparative brightness is given, with the brightest image designated by "1."

[5] Since the index of refraction is typically specified for 589 nm, the calculated index of refraction minimizes the reflections for light of this wavelength.

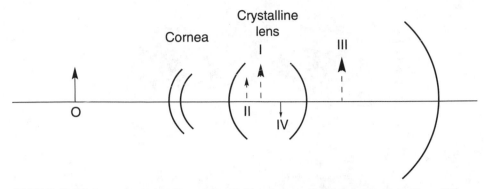

FIGURE 14-12. Approximate locations of the Purkinje images. Purkinje images I, II, III, and IV are formed by the anterior surface of the cornea, posterior surface of the cornea, anterior surface of the lens, and posterior surface of the lens, respectively. All of the images are virtual except for Purkinje image 4, which is formed by the convex posterior surface of the lens.

Purkinje image I has many important clinical applications. It is the image that is used in *keratometry* to determine the corneal radius of curvature (see Fig. 14-20). The first Purkinje image can be utilized to ascertain the *corneal topography* (see Fig. 14-18). When measuring *angle kappa* to determine the amount of eccentric fixation or performing the *Hirschberg test* to measure the angle of strabismus, the clinician views Purkinje image I (Fig. 14-13).

Purkinje image III—the image formed by reflection off the anterior surface of the crystalline lens—changes size during accommodation. During the process of accommodation, the radius of curvature of the anterior lens surface decreases, causing a decrease in the size of the reflected image.

Location of Purkinje Image I

Based on our knowledge of mirrors, we can calculate the location of the first Purkinje image (Fig. 14-14). This image is formed by the anterior surface of the cornea, which has a radius of curvature of 7.80 mm (Gullstrand schematic eye #2). The surface is convex, giving it negative reflective power. We calculate this reflective power as follows:

$$P = -2/r$$
$$P = -2/.0078 \text{ m}$$
$$P = -256.41 \text{ D}$$

Let us assume that the object is at infinity, giving it a vergence of zero. Using the vergence relationship, we have

$$L' = L + P$$
$$L' = 0 - 256.41 \text{ D}$$

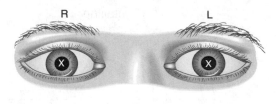

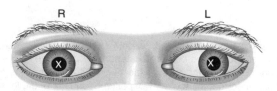

FIGURE 14-13. In the Hirschberg test, the position of Purkinje image I (with respect to the center of the pupil) in one eye is compared to its position in the fellow eye. This test is clinically useful for diagnosing strabismus (an eye turn), particularly in nonresponsive patients. **A.** The patient's two eyes are aligned with the fixation light. As a result, Purkinje image I, which is represented by an *x*, is located in the same position in each eye. **B.** This patient has left eye exotropia—the left eye turns (rotates) outward; consequently, the left eye's Purkinje image is located closer to the nasal edge of the pupil. The rotation of the eye causes Purkinje image I to move with respect to the pupil. The absolute position of the image itself does not significantly move; rather, the eye moves.

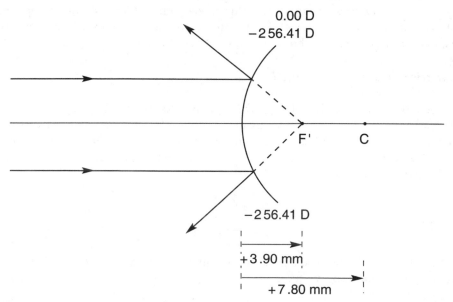

FIGURE 14-14. The vergence relationship can be used to calculate the location of Purkinje image I.

$$L' = -256.41 \text{ D}$$

The image is virtual, and its distance from the corneal surface is

$$L' = -1/l'$$
$$l' = -1/-256.41D$$
$$l' = +0.0039 \text{ m or } +3.90 \text{ mm}$$

Purkinje image I is located 3.90 mm to the right of the corneal surface.

There is another way to approach this problem. Since the object is at infinity, the image is located at the secondary focal point of the mirror. The secondary focal length can be determined from the radius of curvature, as follows:

$$r = 2f'$$
$$+7.80 \text{ mm} = 2f'$$
$$f' = +3.90 \text{ mm}$$

Location of Purkinje Image III

Purkinje image III is formed by reflection off the anterior surface of the crystalline lens. Locating this image is a bit complicated because it is formed by rays that are first refracted by the cornea,[6] then reflected off the anterior surface of the crystalline lens, and then refracted once again by the cornea (Fig. 14-15A). We can simplify the calculations by treating the combined refracting surface and mirror as a single system that we call an *equivalent mirror.*

An equivalent mirror consists of the images of a reflecting surface and its center of curvature as viewed through the *refracting* elements of the system. Purkinje image III is formed by the equivalent mirror that is constituted of the anterior surface of the crystalline lens and its center of curvature, *as viewed through the cornea* (Fig. 14-15B). To construct the equivalent mirror, we consider the anterior surface of the lens as an object and the cornea as a refracting element.[7] The refracting power of the cornea[8] is

$$P = \frac{n' - n}{r}$$

$$P = \frac{1.333 - 1.000}{.0078 \text{ m}}$$

$$P = +42.69 \text{ D}$$

---

[6] For the purposes of this discussion, we treat the cornea as a thin lens.

[7] The cornea can be treated as either a refracting or reflecting element. We are now treating the cornea as a refracting element.

[8] To determine the refracting power of the cornea, we use the Gullstrand eye #2 corneal radius of curvature. We do not use the radius of curvature for the reduced eye because this radius would give us the total refracting power of the eye, combining the powers of both the cornea and lens.

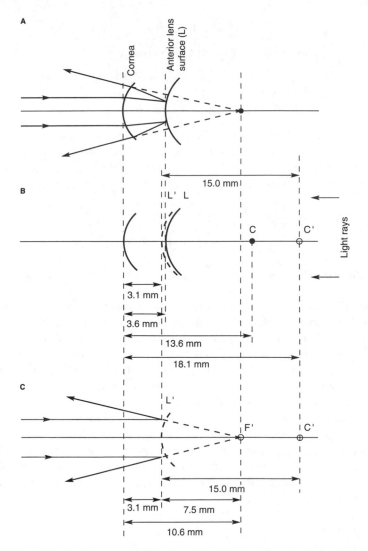

FIGURE 14-15A. Purkinge image III is formed by light rays that are first refracted by the cornea, then reflected off the anterior surface of the lens, and finally refracted again by the cornea. **B.** The equivalent mirror consists of the anterior surface of the crystalline lens and its center of curvature as viewed through the cornea. *L* is the anterior surface of lens, *L'* is the virtual image of the lens surface that is formed by the cornea, *C* is the center of curvature of the anterior surface of the lens, and *C'* is the virtual image of the center of curvature of the anterior lens surface as formed by the cornea. **C.** The equivalent mirror can be used to locate the image that is formed by reflection off the anterior surface of the crystalline lens. The secondary focal point of the equivalent mirror (*F'*) is midway between the surface of the equivalent mirror and its center of curvature. For an object located at infinity, Purkinje image III is located at the secondary focal point of the equivalent mirror. The focal point of the equivalent mirror *cannot* be determined by locating the image of the actual focal point; rather, it must be determined after first locating the equivalent mirror's surface and center of curvature (as we did in the text).

The distance from the anterior lens surface to the cornea is 3.6 mm. This is the object distance (Fig. 14-15B). The object is located in aqueous, and its vergence is[9]

$$|L| = |n / l|$$
$$|L| = |1.333 / .0036 \text{ mm}|$$
$$L = -370.28 \text{ D}$$

Because the object is real, the object vergence has been designated with a minus sign. The vergence relationship is used to locate the image:

$$L' = L + P$$
$$L' = -370.28 \text{ D} + 42.69 \text{ D}$$
$$L' = -327.59 \text{ D}$$

The negative vergence tells us that the image is virtual; a virtual image is located on the same side of the *refracting* element as the object. Since the rays that form the image are located in air, the image distance is

$$|l'| = |n' / L'|$$
$$|l'| = |(1.000)(1000) / -327.59 \text{ D}|$$
$$|l'| = |3.05 \text{ mm}|$$

The surface of the equivalent mirror is 3.1 mm to the right of the cornea.

Next we locate the center of curvature of the equivalent mirror. We treat the center of curvature of the crystalline lens (anterior surface) as an object and the cornea as a refracting element.[10] The object vergence is

$$|L| = |n / l|$$
$$|L| = |1.333 / .0136 \text{ mm}|$$
$$L = -98.01 \text{ D}$$

This object vergence has been designated as negative because the object is real. To locate the image, we use the vergence relationship

$$L' = L + P$$
$$L' = -98.01 \text{ D} + 42.69 \text{ D}$$
$$L' = -55.32 \text{ D}$$

---

[9] The object (anterior surface of the crystalline lens) is located to the right of the refracting surface; its image is formed by light that travels from right to left. Because our linear sign convention does not apply to light traveling from right to left, we have used the absolute values of the linear distances to calculate vergence. Alternatively, we can reverse the diagram so that the anterior lens surface is located to the left of the cornea. See Figure 14-16 for this alternative solution.

[10] The distance from the cornea to the center of curvature of the crystalline lens anterior surface is 13.6 mm (Gullstrand eye #2).

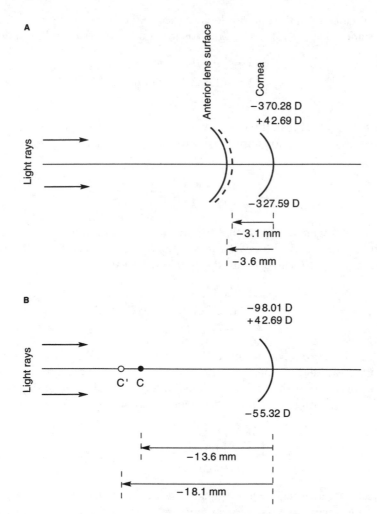

FIGURE 14-16. Another way to locate the images of the anterior lens surface and its center of curvature is to use our linear sign convention. To do so, light must travel from left to right. We have redrawn the eye so that the objects (the anterior lens surface and its center of curvature) are to the left of the cornea. **A.** Location of the image of the anterior lens surface. **B.** Location of image of the center of curvature of the anterior lens surface.

This negative image vergence tells us that the image is virtual and located on the same side of the cornea as the object. The refracted rays that form the image are located in air:

$$|l'| = |n'/L'|$$
$$|l'| = |1.000(1000)/-55.32 \text{ D}|$$
$$|l'| = |18.08 \text{ mm}|$$

The center of curvature of the equivalent lens is located 18.1 mm to the right of the corneal surface.

By examining Figure 14-15B, we see that the center of curvature of the equivalent mirror is 15.0 mm to the right of its surface (18.1 mm − 3.1 mm = 15.0 mm). Therefore the radius of curvature of the equivalent mirror is 15.0 mm. The focal length of the equivalent mirror is 7.5 mm (it is half of the radius of curvature).[11]

The equivalent mirror can be considered to have the properties of a typical mirror. If the object is located at infinity, the image is located at the focal point of the equivalent mirror, which is 7.5 mm beyond the surface of the equivalent mirror (Fig. 14-15C). Since the surface of the equivalent mirror is 3.1 mm to the right of the corneal surface, the image—Purkinje image III—is 10.6 mm to the right of the actual corneal surface.

CORNEAL TOPOGRAPHY [12]

For the purposes of fitting contact lenses, evaluating the cornea prior to and following surgical or laser refractive procedures, and diagnosing certain conditions (e.g., keratoconus[13]), it is important to know the topography of the cornea. Contrary to the schematic eyes that we have considered thus far, the cornea is actually an *aspherical*, not a spherical, structure: it does not have a single radius of curvature (Fig. 14-17). Rather, the center (i.e., paraxial region) of the cornea is more curved than is its periphery.[14]

---

[11] In deriving the equivalent mirror, it is necessary to first locate the images of the reflecting surface (the equivalent lens surface) and center of curvature (the equivalent center of curvature) and then to calculate the focal length. *The equivalent focal point cannot be directly determined by locating the image of a surface's focal point.*

[12] The remaining material in this chapter emphasizes astigmatism. You may wish to review Chapter 9 before reading on.

[13] *Keratoconus* is a degenerative corneal disease in which the central cornea becomes progressively steeper and thinner. It is treated with custom rigid contact lenses and/or penetrating keratoplasty.

[14] As we will learn in Chapter 15, the flattening of the periphery of the cornea reduces the eye's spherical aberration.

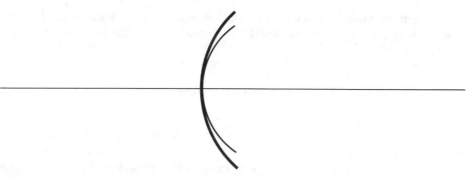

FIGURE 14-17. The cornea does not have a single radius of curvature—it is aspherical. The center (axial region) of the cornea is more curved than its periphery (paraxial region). The light curve represents a spherical surface and the darker curve, an aspherical surface.

Certain *corneal topographers*—clinical instruments that are used to determine the shape of the cornea—utilize Purkinje image I. Lighted rings of known diameters are reflected off the cornea. The dimensions of each of these rings are compared to the dimensions of its reflected image (Fig. 14-18). Using this information, the topographer calculates the radii of curvature of the cornea from its center to its periphery to construct a *topographic map*. Figure 14-19 shows additional examples of corneal topographic maps.

KERATOMETRY AND CONTACT LENSES

For certain clinical applications, it is not necessary to obtain a detailed topographic map of the cornea. In *keratometry,* the radii of curvature for the two principal meridians are determined at a given corneal eccentricity.[15] The dimensions of lighted objects—known as *mires*—are compared with the dimensions of their reflected corneal images, thereby allowing the determination of the radii of curvature of the principal meridians (Fig. 14-20). Assuming an index of refraction of 1.3375, which is the index of refraction of the tear film, the keratometer converts these radii to dioptric values.

Corneal keratometry readings (frequently called *K readings*) are often used in the fitting of corneal contact lenses. By convention, laboratories typically convert the curvature of the back surface of the contact lens—*the base curve*—to dioptric units. In making this conversion, the index of refraction of the tears, not the index of refraction of the contact lens material, is used.

Let us discuss a few examples in which rigid contact lenses are used to correct ametropia. This discussion will serve as an introduction to the optics of con-

---

[15] The two principal meridians, which are orthogonal to each other, are the cornea's most curved and least curved meridians (Chap. 9).

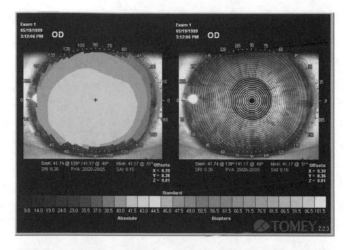

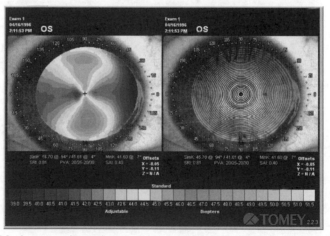

FIGURE 14-18A. A commonly used corneal topographer works by shining lighted rings of known dimensions onto the cornea and measuring the dimensions of the reflected image (i.e., Purkinje image I on the right panel). The topography of the cornea is displayed on a color-coded map, using blue to represent flatter areas and reds to indicate steeper areas. In this black-and-white rendition of a corneal topography map, steepness is indicated by shades of gray (left panel). This cornea does not have significant astigmatism—it is spherical. **B.** Topographic map of a cornea of a patient with with-the-rule astigmatism. Although Purkinje image I looks normal, the topographic map reveals that the vertical meridian of the eye is steeper than the horizontal meridan. *(Illustrations courtesy of the Tomey Corporation USA.)*

tact lenses; it is not intended to be comprehensive or detailed. *Consider a rigid contact lens with a base curve of 42.00 D that sits on a nonastigmatic cornea. The K readings are*

43.00/90

43.00/180

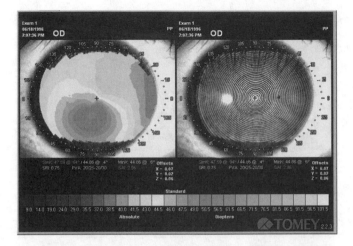

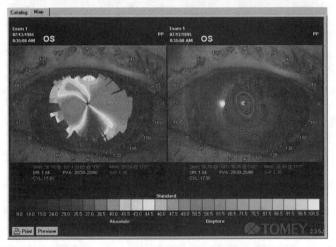

FIGURE 14-19A. Topographic map of a keratoconic cornea. Note the steep apex (which is not in the center of the cornea). **B.** Following penetrating keratoplasty, the cornea shows marked asymmetries.

The patient's prescription when measured at the corneal plane is −3.00 DS. If the power of the contact lens is −2.00 DS, will it correct the patient's ametropia? Yes, it will! This is because the base curve of the contact lens is flatter than the cornea, creating a so-called *fluid lens* that has a power of −1.00 DS (Fig.14-21A).

The anterior surface of this fluid lens has the same curvature as the contact lens's base curve. The fluid lens, which is composed of tears, has an index of refraction of 1.3375. The anterior surface of the fluid lens has a power of +42.00 DS (equal to the base curve of the contact lens). The posterior surface of the fluid lens has the same curvature as the cornea. Again assuming an index of 1.3375, the power of the posterior surface of the fluid lens is −43.00 DS. Consequently, the

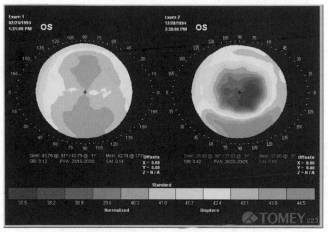

FIGURE 14-19C. The left panel shows a cornea before photorefractive surgery; the right panel shows the cornea following the surgery. Note the extreme flatness of the central cornea following the procedure. (*Illustrations courtesy of Tomey Corporation USA.*)

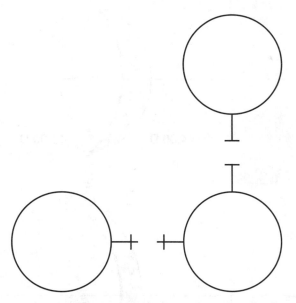

FIGURE 14-20. In keratometry, these lighted objects (called *mires*) are reflected off the cornea. Since the dimensions of the mires are known, the radius of curvature of the cornea can be calculated at the eccentricity of the cornea on which the mires fall.

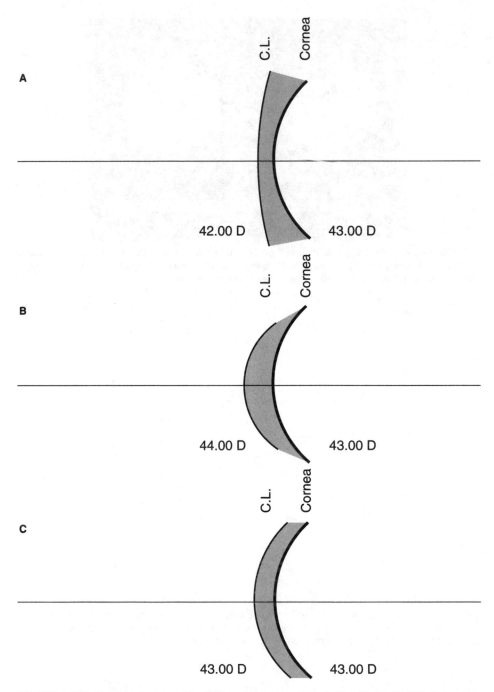

FIGURE 14-21. Fluid lenses formed by rigid contact lenses (CL). **A.** The CL (42.00 D) is flatter than the cornea (43.00 D), creating a −1.00 DS fluid lens. **B.** The CL (44.00 D) is steeper than the cornea (43.00 D), creating a +1.00 DS fluid lens. **C.** The CL (43.00 D) is the same curvature as the cornea (43.00 D), creating a fluid lens of zero power.

fluid lens has a power of −1.00 DS. The combination of the −2.00 DS contact lens and the −1.00-DS fluid lens fully corrects the 3.00 D myope.

What power contact lens would be required to correct this 3.00 D myope if the contact lens has a base curve of 44.00 D? Figure 14-21B shows that the fluid lens has a power of +1.00 DS. Therefore, to correct the myopia, the contact lens must have a power of −4.00 DS. *What power would be required to correct this myope if the contact lens has a base curve of 43.00 D?* Since the anterior and posterior surfaces of the fluid lens have the same curvature, the fluid lens has no power (Fig.14-21C). Therefore, a −3.00 DS contact lens is required.

Let us consider another example. *A patient's right eye has the following K readings and refraction as determined as the corneal plane:*

$$44.00/90$$
$$43.00/180$$
$$-5.00 = -1.00 \times 180$$

A rigid contact lens with a base curve of 43.00 D is fitted to this cornea (i.e., fitted on flat K*). Using the terminology of Chapter 9, diagnose the patient's refractive error. What is the power of the contact lens required to correct the patient's ametropia?*

First, draw a cross that shows the prescription (i.e., the required correction) and a cross that shows the patient's corneal powers (i.e., K readings) (Fig. 14-22A). The former illustrates that the vertical meridian of the eye is more powerful than the horizontal meridian. The patient has compound myopic with-the-rule astigmatism. The K readings tell us that the cornea is the source of the astigmatism (rather than the crystalline lens). A cornea that has cylindrical power is said to be *toric*.

If the base curve of the contact lens is 43.00 D, what is the power of the fluid lens? From Figure 14-22B, we see that fluid lens has a power of −1.00 D in its vertical meridian and no power in its horizontal meridian. Therefore, a −5.00 DS contact lens in combination with the fluid lens will fully correct the refractive error.

If the contact lens has a base curve of 44.00 D, what power is required to correct the ametropia? The fluid lens has powers of zero in the vertical meridian and +1.00 D in the horizontal meridian (Figure 14-22C). Consequently, a −6.00 DS contact lens will correct the ametropia.

JAVAL'S RULE

The cornea and crystalline lens are the primary sources of ocular astigmatism. Corneal toricity can be directly measured with a keratometer or corneal topographer. When the K readings are known, the total amount of ocular astigmatism as measured in the spectacle plane can be estimated using *Javal's rule*:

Est. ocular astig. = (corneal toricity)(1.25) + (−0.50 DC × 090)

where *Est. ocular astig.* = the estimated ocular astigmatism in the spectacle plane

Corneal toricity = the *correction* for corneal cylindrical power in minus cylinder form (as measured in the corneal plane)

A   Prescription

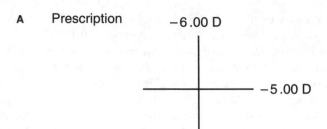

K reading

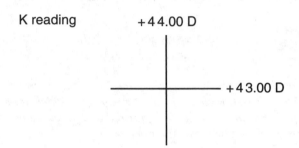

B   Fluid lens

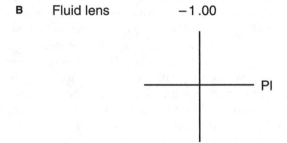

C   Fluid lens

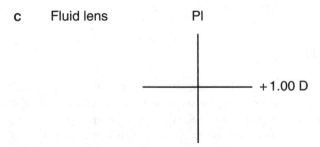

FIGURE 14-22A. The prescription and corneal power of the cornea discussed in the text. **B.** Fluid lens when this cornea is fitted with a contact lens with a base curve of 43.00 D. **C.** Fluid lens when this cornea is fitted with a contact lens that has a base curve of 44.00 D.

Javal's rule assumes an average crystalline lens astigmatism (*lenticular astigmatism*) of −0.50 DC × 090. To correct for lens effectivity, the corneal toricity is multiplied by a factor of 1.25.

Let us look at an example. A patient's K's are as follows:

43.00/090

44.00/180

Based on Javal's rule, what is the estimated ocular astigmatism as measured in the spectacle plane? Figure 14-23A shows the corneal powers on a lens cross. The required cylindrical correction is also given (in minus cylinder form). Javal's rule is applied in Figure 14-23B, resulting in a predicted ocular astigmatism at the spectacle plane of −1.75 DC × 090.

Clinically, Javal's rule is of limited utility because the amount of lenticular astigmatism varies from patient to patient. Although Javal's rule cannot accurately predict the ocular astigmatism for an individual patient, it does reinforce the important point that lenticular astigmatism is often against-the-rule. The amount of against-the-rule astigmatism tends to increase with age due to changes in the crystalline lens.

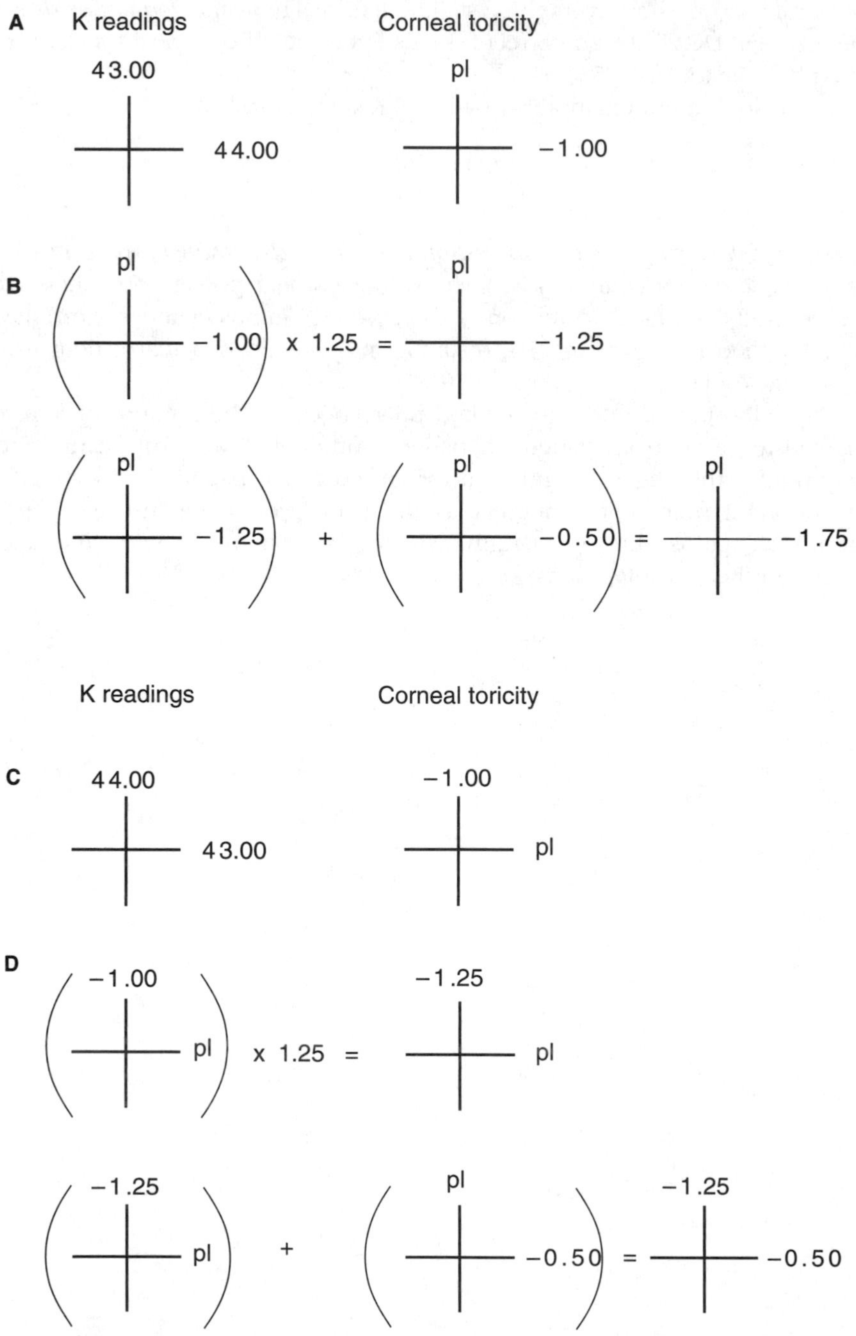

A   K readings   Corneal toricity

43.00   pl

$+$ 44.00 $+$ −1.00

B

$\left(\begin{array}{c} pl \\ + \\ \end{array} -1.00 \right)$ x 1.25 = $\begin{array}{c} pl \\ + \\ \end{array}$ −1.25

$\left(\begin{array}{c} pl \\ + \\ \end{array} -1.25 \right)$ + $\left(\begin{array}{c} pl \\ + \\ \end{array} -0.50 \right)$ = $\begin{array}{c} pl \\ + \\ \end{array}$ −1.75

K readings   Corneal toricity

C   44.00   −1.00

$+$ 43.00 $+$ pl

D

$\left(\begin{array}{c} -1.00 \\ + \\ \end{array} pl \right)$ x 1.25 = $\begin{array}{c} -1.25 \\ + \\ \end{array}$ pl

$\left(\begin{array}{c} -1.25 \\ + \\ \end{array} pl \right)$ + $\left(\begin{array}{c} pl \\ + \\ \end{array} -0.50 \right)$ = $\begin{array}{c} -1.25 \\ + \\ \end{array}$ −0.50

FIGURE 14-23A. K readings and the corneal toricity for the example discussed in the text. **B.** Application of Javal's rule to estimate the amount of ocular astigmatism. **C.** Another example that shows how Javal's rule can be used to estimate the amount of ocular astigmatism. The K readings are 44.00 D/090 and 43.00 D/180. **D.** Calculation of estimated ocular astigmatism.

P Self-Assessment Problems

1. An object is located 5.00 cm anterior to a mirror that has a radius of curvature of −30.00 cm. (a) Locate the image. (b) Is the image real or virtual? (c) If the object is 2.00 cm in height, what is the height of the image?

2. An object is located 25.00 cm anterior to a mirror that has a focal length of +15.00 cm. Answer the questions asked in Problem 1.

3. A real image is located 40.00 cm from a +30.00 D mirror. Locate the object.

4. A virtual image is located 10.00 cm from a −30.00 D mirror. Locate the object.

5. An object is located 20.00 cm anterior to a +15.00 D lens. This lens is located 3.00 cm anterior to a mirror that has a radius of curvature of +2.00 cm. (a) Locate the image. (b) What is the magnification of the optical system?

6. A circular light is located 10.00 cm anterior to the cornea of the eye. Assuming that the anterior surface of the cornea has a radius of 7.80 mm, locate the first Purkinje image.

7. A circular light is located 7.00 cm anterior to the cornea of the eye. If the first Purkinje image is oval in shape with its long axis vertical, is the corneal astigmatism with-the-rule or against-the-rule?

8. A patient' keratometry readings and refractive error (right eye) are as follows:

$$42.00 \text{ D}/90$$
$$44.00 \text{ D}/180$$
$$+2.00 = +2.00 \times 180$$

Is the corneal astigmatism with-the-rule or against-the-rule?

9. (a) What percentage of light is reflected by the front surface of a lens that is made from a high-index material ($n = 1.62$)? (b) Answer the same question for a plastic lens. (c) For which lens would an antireflection coating be most important? Why? (d) What should be the index of refraction of the antireflection coating for the higher-index lens?

10. An eye has the following spectacle refractive error and keratometry readings:

$$-3.00 = -1.50 \times 180$$
$$43.50 \text{ D}/90$$
$$42.00 \text{ D}/180$$

(a) The eye is fit with a rigid contact lens that has a base curve of 42.00 D. To fully correct the refractive error, what should be the power of the (b) If the contact lens has a base curve of 43.00 D, what power is required to fully correct the eye? (c) If the eye is fit with a contact lens that has a power of -2.50 DS, what base curve is required to correct the eye?

11. A cornea has the following K readings:

$$41.00/090$$
$$43.00/180$$

Use Javal's rule to estimate the amount of ocular astigmatism as measured in the spectacle plane.

12. After taking corneal Ks and applying Javal's rule, you estimate the ocular astigmatic correction in the spectacle plane to be $-5.00 \text{ DC} \times 090$. (a) If the vertical meridian has a K of 44.00, what is the K of the horizontal meridian? (b) Is the corneal toricity with-the-rule or against-the-rule?

Aberrations

15

Optical aberrations degrade the image formed by an optical system. Certain of these aberrations occur with monochromatic light (*monochromatic aberrations*), while others occur only in polychromatic light (*chromatic aberrations*).

THE PARAXIAL ASSUMPTION

The paraxial equation (i.e., vergence relationship) is very useful because it allows us to readily locate the images produced by spherical optical systems. In the derivation of the paraxial equation, however, an assumption is made that limits its predictive powers. Let us derive the paraxial equation so that we can become familiar with this assumption.

Figure 15-1 shows a light ray incident upon a spherical refracting surface. According to Snell's law,

$$n\sin\theta = n'\sin\theta'$$

By definition, paraxial rays make small angles at the lens.[1] For these rays, we can make the assumption that $\sin\theta = \theta$ (where θ is in radians). Snell's law is then rewritten as

$$n\theta = n'\theta'$$

From Figure 15-1, we see that

$$\theta = \alpha + \beta$$
$$\beta = \theta' + \delta$$

or

$$\theta' = \beta - \delta$$

---

[1]Paraxial rays are close to the optical axis of the lens and are incident on the central area of the lens.

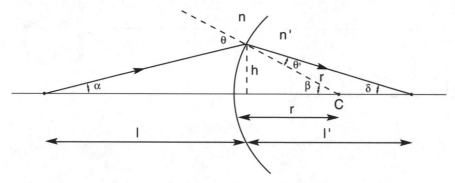

FIGURE 15-1. Snell's law can be used to derive the paraxial relationship. This relationship is accurate only for paraxial rays.

Substituting into Snell's law, we have

$$n(\alpha + \beta) = n'(\beta - \delta)$$

or

$$n'\delta = -n\alpha + \beta(n' - n)$$

But from Figure 15-1, we see that

$$\alpha = h/-l$$
$$\beta = h/r$$

and

$$\delta = h/l'$$

By substitution, we have the paraxial equation

$$n'/l' = n/l + (n' - n)/r$$

or

$$L' = L + P$$

SEIDEL ABERRATIONS

For small angles, the assumption that $\sin\theta = \theta$ is reasonable. It is not accurate, however, for larger angles. A better estimate of $\sin\theta$ is given by the following expansion:

$$\sin\theta = \theta - (\theta^3/3!) + (\theta^5/5!) - (\theta^7/7!) + \dots$$

When the third order approximation $(\theta - \theta^3 / 3!)$ is used, we find five different ways in which there are deviations from the paraxial equation. These interrelated deviations are referred to as *Seidel aberrations (or classic aberrations)*. The five aberrations are spherical aberration, coma, radial astigmatism, curvature of field, and distortion. (As discussed later in this chapter, it is now common to characterize aberrations in terms of Zernike polynomials.)

Because of these aberrations, the image formed by a *spherical* optical system is not perfect. Ophthalmic lenses are generally designed so that certain of the aberrations are minimized.

Spherical Aberration

In *spherical aberration*, light rays that strike the center of a lens (i.e., the paraxial region of the lens) are focused in a different plane than the light rays that strike the periphery of the lens (i.e., the nonparaxial region of the lens). This aberration can take two basic forms: *positive (undercorrected)* spherical aberration and *negative (overcorrected)* spherical aberration. In positive spherical aberration, the rays that strike the nonparaxial region of the lens are focused closer to the lens than are the paraxial rays (Fig. 15-2A). When the paraxial rays are focused nearest the lens, we have negative spherical aberration (Fig. 15-2B).

Spherical lenses manifest positive spherical aberration. For both plus and minus spherical lenses, the nonparaxial rays are more refracted than the paraxial rays (Fig. 15-3). As the diameter of the bundle of rays striking a lens increases, the amount of the spherical aberration increases. Consequently, the amount of spherical aberration can be reduced by positioning a small-diameter aperture in close proximity to the lens (either in front of or behind the lens) (Fig. 15-4).

Spherical aberration has both a longitudinal and a lateral (transverse) expression (Fig. 15-5). *Longitudinal spherical aberration* is the distance between the paraxial and nonparaxial foci as measured along the optical axis. In comparison, *lateral spherical aberration* is the distance between the paraxial and nonparaxial rays as measured at a given point along the optical axis.

The amount of spherical aberration present in an image is dependent on, among other factors, the radii of curvatures of the front and back surfaces of the lens. The lens radii of curvature are used to calculate the so-called *bending factor*,[2] X:

$$X = (r_2 + r_1) / (r_2 - r_1)$$

Where

---

[2] The bending factor is sometimes called the *shape factor*, but it should not be confused with the shape factor in Chapter 13. The latter is applicable to magnification, not spherical aberration.

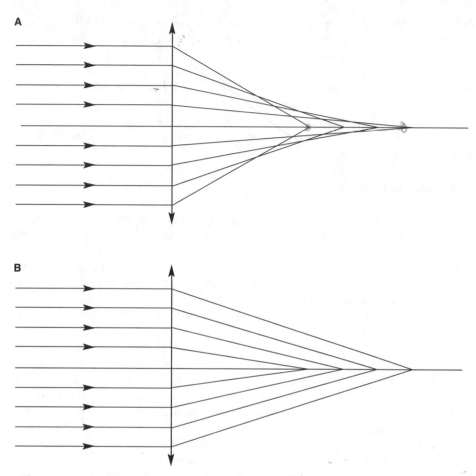

FIGURE 15-2A. Positive (undercorrected) spherical aberration. **B.** Negative (overcorrected) spherical aberration.

r_1 = the radius of curvature of the anterior lens surface
r_2 = the radius of curvature of the posterior lens surface

As the value of X decreases, the amount of spherical aberration becomes less.

Figure 15-6A shows spherical aberration plotted as a function of the bending factor. Included in the plot are diagrams of lenses that have various bending factors—the lenses appear to be bent in different ways. As you can see, spherical aberration is minimized for lenses that have an approximately planoconvex shape.

The side of the lens that faces the incoming rays is critical in determining the amount of spherical aberration. For the lenses in Figure 15-6A, light rays are assumed to travel from the left to the right. To minimize spherical aberrations with, for example, a planoconvex lens that is used to correct hyperopia, the convex side should face the incoming rays (i.e., it should be the front surface) (Fig. 15-6B).

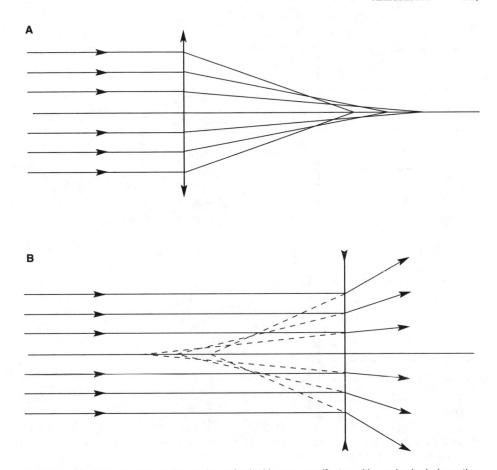

FIGURE 15-3. Both positive and negative spherical lenses manifest positive spherical aberration.

Even with an optimal bending factor, spherical aberration can be significant. This is particularly the case with high-power ophthalmic lenses. *Aspheric* surfaces can be used to minimize spherical aberrations. Whereas the surface of a spherical lens has a single radius of curvature, the surface of an aspheric lens has many different radii of curvature (Fig. 15-7). In an aspheric plus lens, the radius of curvature increases as we go from the center of the lens to its periphery. That is, the periphery of the lens becomes flatter to compensate for positive spherical aberration.

Coma

Figure 15-8 shows the image that is formed when a bundle of light rays from an off-axis point source strike a spherical plus lens. The image is not a point; rather, it is comet-shaped. This aberration—*coma*—occurs because the peripheral rays

A

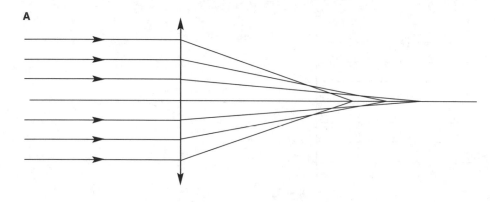

B

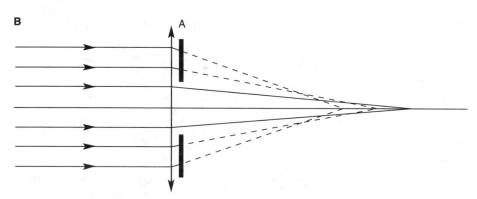

FIGURE 15-4. An aperture (A) that decreases the diameter of the bundle of rays decreases the amount of spherical aberration.

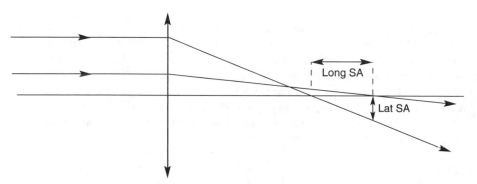

FIGURE 15-5. Spherical aberration has both a longitudinal (*long SA*) and lateral (transverse) expression (*lat SA*).

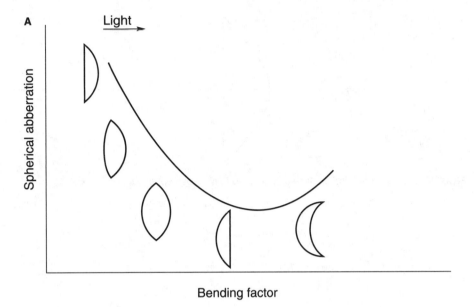

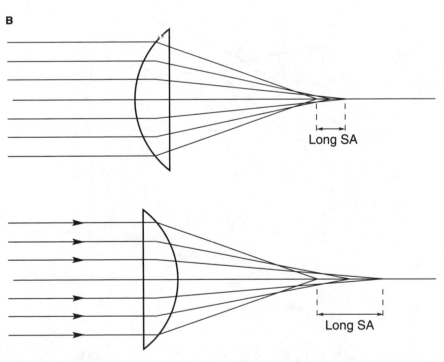

FIGURE 15-6A. Spherical aberration as a function of the bending factor. **B.** For a planoconvex lens, spherical aberration is minimized when light rays are incident on the convex surface of the lens.

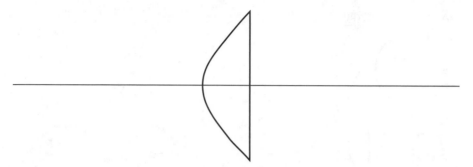

FIGURE 15-7. An aspherical surface can be used to minimize spherical aberration.

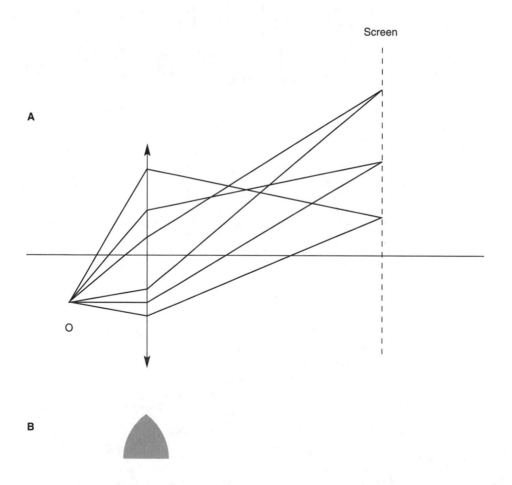

FIGURE 15-8A. Coma results when an off-axis point source is imaged by a spherical lens. **B.** Coma pattern seen on the screen in **A.**

of an off-axis ray bundle are more refracted than the central rays of the bundle; the peripheral rays are focused closer to the optical axis than are the central rays. The resulting image has a comet-like shape.

It is often stated that coma occurs only for off-axis objects. This is true for optical systems in which the optical components are centered and not tilted with respect to each other. Coma can, however, occur for an optical system such as the eye, where the optical components are noncentered and tilted with respect to each other. Indeed, coma is a major foveal aberration.

Like spherical aberration, coma increases as the diameter of the ray pencil increases. If an aperture is placed close to a lens and the diameter of the aperture is decreased, the amount of coma and spherical aberration decreases. An optical system free of both coma and spherical aberration is said to be *aplanat-*

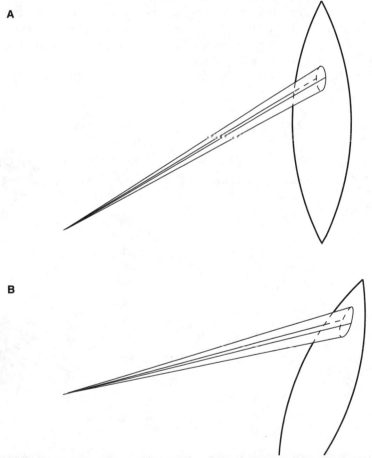

A

B

FIGURE 15-9. Radial astigmatism can occur **(A)** when light rays from an off-axis point source strike the periphery of a spherical lens or **(B)** when light rays from an on-axis point source strike a spherical lens that is tilted.

ic. It is relatively easy to correct for coma in thin ophthalmic lenses. The coma of a thin lens is trivial compared to that of the eye.

Radial Astigmatism

We can think of a point source as emitting both horizontally and vertically diverging light rays (see Chap. 9). If the point source is on the optical axis of a spherical lens, the angle of incidence for the horizontally diverging rays is equal to the angle of incidence for the vertically diverging rays. If the point source is off-axis however, the horizontally diverging rays strike the surface of the lens at a different angle than the vertically diverging rays (i.e., the rays strike the lens obliquely) (Fig. 15-9A). This results in *radial astigmatism* (also called *oblique* or *marginal astigmatism*). The same effect can occur for an object that is on the optical axis, if the lens is tilted with respect to this axis (Fig. 15-9B).

Clinically, radial astigmatism can occur when a patient views objects that are not on the optical axis of his or her corrective lens. Consider Figure 15-10A, which shows a patient wearing spectacle lenses that have a *pantoscopic angle* of zero—the lenses are not tilted with respect to the frontal plane of the patient's face. When the patient views a distant object that is along the lens's optical axis,

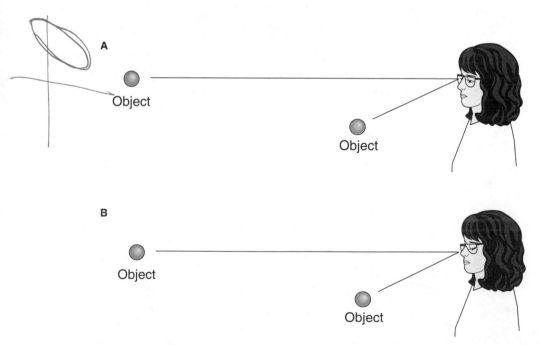

FIGURE 15-10A. If the pantoscopic angle is zero, there is no radial astigmatism when the patient views a distant on-axis object. Radial astigmatism is present, however, when he or she views a near object. **B.** Increasing the pantoscopic angle reduces the radial astigmatism present when viewing a near object but increases the radial astigmatism when viewing a distant object.

there is no radial astigmatism. Radial astigmatism does occur, however, when the patient views an off-axis near object through these spectacle lenses. The lenses are tilted with respect to the near object.[3]

The amount of radial astigmatism induced by viewing a near object can be reduced if the corrective lenses are less tilted with respect to the near object. This is accomplished by increasing the pantoscopic angle of the corrective lenses (as shown in Fig. 15-10B). Doing so, however, causes radial astigmatism to be introduced when the patient views distant objects. While no single pantoscopic angle can eliminate marginal astigmatism for all viewing angles, it is a factor that should be taken into account in prescribing and dispensing ophthalmic lenses. As the spherical power of the corrective lens increases, radial astigmatism becomes more pronounced.

Curvature of Field

Not all points on the extended object in Figure 15-11 are the same distance from the spherical converging lens. The tip and base of the arrow are further from the lens (the object distance is l_2) than the center of the object (the object distance is l_1). Consequently, the image distances for the tip and base of the arrow are

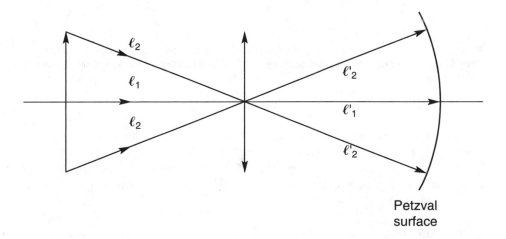

FIGURE 15-11. The image plane for a flat object is curved, resulting in curvature of field. Curvature of field occurs because the off-axis portions of the object (the tip and base of the arrow) are further from the lens (object distance of l_2) than the on-axis portions (object distance of l_1). Consequently, the image distance is less for the tip and base of the arrow (l'_2) than for the on-axis portion of the arrow (l'_1).

---

[3] This assumes that the patient turns her eyes to view the near object rather than tilting her head.

Grid object

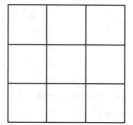

Barrel
distortion

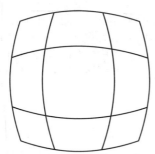

Pincushion
distortion

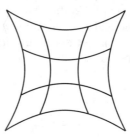

FIGURE 15-12. When viewed through a spherical lens, a grid pattern can appear distorted. Barrel distortion can occur with minus spherical lenses (left), while pincushion distortion is found with plus spherical lenses.

less than for the center of the arrow. The result is an image plane that is not flat, but is curved[4]—this is referred to as *curvature of field.*

Off-axis rays that pass through the center of a lens can cause curvature of field. For this reason, a small aperature placed close to the lens may not eliminate this aberration.

Distortion

The lateral magnification in the center of a spherical lens is different than the lateral magnification in the periphery the lens. For an extended source, this results in distortion. There are two basic types of distortion: *barrel distortion,* which is generally found with minus lenses, and *pincushion distortion,* which is generally found with plus lenses (Fig. 15 12).

---

[4] This curved image plane is sometimes called a *Petzval surface.*

SPHERICAL ABERRATION OF THE HUMAN EYE

As more of the nonparaxial region of an optical system—including the human eye—is exposed to light rays, optical aberrations increase. When the pupil is about 3 mm or less, as it may be under daylight conditions, the eye manifests insignificant optical aberrations.[5]

Since we typically align the visual axis of our eye with the object we wish to view, spherical aberration is of considerable concern.[6] The unaccommodated eye typically (but not always) manifests positive spherical aberration, which tends to increase with age (Guirao et al., 2000). The positive spherical aberration would be even greater if not for the aspherical nature of the cornea—the periphery of the cornea is flatter than its center (Chap. 9).

As the eye accommodates, the amount of positive spherical aberration decreases; it is minimized when the eye accommodates about 1.5 D. Further accommodation results in increasing amounts of negative spherical aberration (Ivanoff, 1956).

Spherical aberration may have clinical implications for nighttime vision. Under dim lighting conditions the pupil dilates, exposing the retina to nonparaxial light rays. These light rays may be focused in front of the retina, making the eye myopic. This can be one contributing factor to *night myopia*—myopia that is present only when the illumination is low.[7] Clinically, consideration should be given to prescribing lenses with slightly more minus power (or less plus power) for those patients who do considerable nighttime driving.

WAVEFRONT SENSING AND ADAPTIVE OPTICS

The eye's monochromatic aberrations can degrade the image that is focused on the retina and thereby limit a patient's ability to resolve detail. If these aberrations could be corrected, it may be possible to improve vision from the typical 20/20 or 20/15 to something like 20/10.

Monochromatic aberrations also limit the clinician's ability to examine a patient's fundus.[8] Even if we could fully compensate for the aberrations present in the doctor's eye, the fundus must still be viewed through the optics of the patient's eye. The optical aberrations in the patient's eye degrade the image that

---

[5] As the pupil decreases in diameter, diffraction—not aberrations—limits the image quality (see Chap. 11).

[6] Curiously, the *optical axis of the eye*, which goes through the centers of curvature of the eye's optical elements, and the *visual axis*, which connects the object of regard and the fovea, are not aligned.

[7] The major cause of night myopia appears to be empty-field accommodation. Note that some eyes have negative spherical aberration, not positive spherical aberration.

[8] The fundus consists of the retina and other posterior ocular structures as seen with an ophthalmoscope or biomicroscope.

is seen by the clinican, thereby limiting the clinician's ability to resolve the detail of the fundus. If it were feasible to compensate for the aberrations in the patient's eye, it might then be possible to detect and diagnose certain diseases earlier (i.e., before they would have been apparent on examining the fundus through the eye's aberrations).

In recent years, there has been a heightened interest in the measurement and possible correction of the eye's monochromatic aberrations. The aberrations are measured by determining how much a wavefront of light is distorted by the optics of the eye. This is accomplished with so-called *wavefront sensing devices*.

Measurement of the Eye's Monochromatic Aberrations

The eye's monochromatic aberrations can be measured using devices called aberrometers. Perhaps the most widely discussed such device is the *Hartmann-Shack aberrometer* (Liang et al., 1994). This device focuses a point of light on the retina. The point of light, in turn, serves as an object—a point source—that emits light rays. These light rays travel back out through the eye's optical system, forming a pattern that reveals the eye's monochromatic aberrations.

Let us discuss this in more detail.[9] Figure 15-13A shows the basic design of the Hartmann-Shack aberrometer. If an eye has no aberrations (i.e., a perfect eye), the rays that are emitted by the retinal point source emerge from the eye parallel to each other. These parallel light rays are incident upon an array consisting of many tiny lenslets. The lenslets focus the parallel light rays onto a sensor, forming a regular grid of points (Fig. 15-13B). Each point is aligned with the optical axis of a lenset.

The pattern formed by an actual eye is not a regular grid because the eye has aberrations. As can be seen in Figure 15-13C, the rays that emerge from a normal eye are not perfectly parallel to each other. As a result, the pattern formed by the lenslets is not a regular grid. The manner is which the pattern deviates from a regular grid reveals the nature of the eye's aberrations and can be analyzed to provide a quantitative measure of the eye's various aberrations. When analyzed in this fashion, deviations from a regular grid pattern can be expressed as *Zernike polynomials* (i.e., second order, third order, etc.). It is now common to characterize the aberrations present in an optical system in terms of Zernike polynomials rather than as Seidel aberrations. Table 15-1 gives some of the Zernike polynomials and the equivalent Seidel aberrations.

There is another way to conceptualize the nonparallel light rays in Figure 15-13C. Recall from Chapter 1 that light rays are perpendicular to wavefronts. As can be seen in Figure 15-14A, a point source produces wavefronts that become flatter as they move further away from the source. When a wavefront is infinitely

---

[9] For a more detailed and very lucid description of the Hartmann-Shack aberrometer, see Thibos (2000).

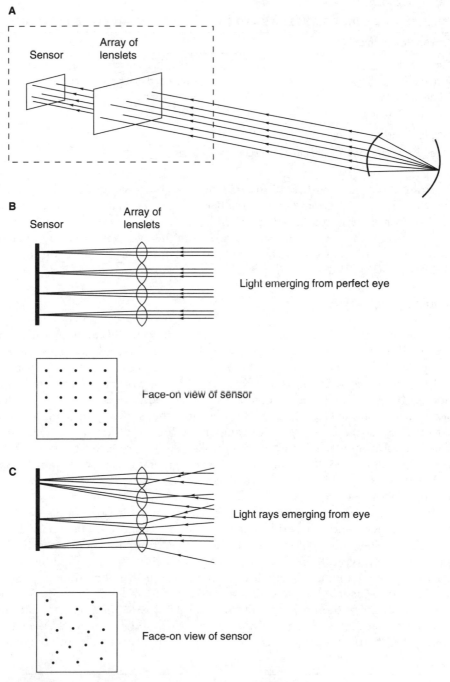

FIGURE 15-13A. Basic design of the Hartmann-Shack aberrometer. The portion of the aberrometer enclosed by the dashed lines is illustrated in more detail in **B** and **C**. **B.** Lenslets focus the parallel light rays that emerge from an eye without aberrations (a perfect eye) onto a sensor, forming a regular grid of points. **C.** Because of aberrations, the rays that actually emerge from the eye do not form a regular grid pattern.

TABLE 15-1. ZERNIKE POLYNOMIALS AND THEIR SEIDEL ABERRATION EQUIVALENTS

Zernike Polynomial[a]	Siedel Aberration
Second order	Ametropia (defocus and astigmatism)
Third order	Coma and other aberrations
Fourth order	Spherical and other aberrations
Fifth to tenth orders	Irregular aberrations[b]

[a] Liang and Williams (1997).

[b] Irregular aberrations are not present in spherical surfaces.

far from a source, it is flat. (Consequently the light rays are parallel to each other.) This flat wavefront forms a regular grid on the Hartmann-Shack wavefront sensor as indicated in Figure 15-14B.

What does the wavefront that emerges from the eye look like? Due to aberrations, the wavefront emerges distorted and/or irregular, forming an irregular grid pattern (Fig. 15-14C).

Supernormal Vision

When a person's pupil is greater than 3 mm in diameter, aberrations can interfere with his or her ability to resolve detail (Liang and Williams, 1997). Compensation for the eye's aberrations results in improved contrast sensitivity and increased resolution, a condition referred to as *supernormal vision*. In the laboratory, it is possible to compensate for aberrations with a so-called *deformable mirror* (Fig. 15-15). By adjusting the surface topography of a deformable mirror, it is possible to compensate for the distortions in the wavefront, thereby minimizing the aberrations—a process referred to as *adaptive optics*.[10] Liang et al (1997) demonstrated that a grating of 55 cycles per degree, which was not visible under normal conditions, was visible when viewed through adaptive optics.

It is conceivable that custom contact lenses or laser procedures, such as PRK or LASIK, could be used to improve vision beyond the customary 20/20 or 20/15 (Applegate, 2000). Laser procedures as normally performed at this time, however, typically increase the eye's monochromatic aberrations rather than decreasing them. Nonetheless, with newer instrumentation, it is now possible to measure the eye's aberrations prior to the laser procedure and then to customize the ablation pattern.[11] The goal is to minimize the aberrations introduced by the laser procedure or to even reduce the aberrations to a level lower than before the procedure. While this is conceivable, the long-term

---

[10] Not only the Seidel aberrations (which are spherical) but also nonspherical (i.e., *irregular*) aberrations can be corrected.

[11] The eye's total aberrations are a combination of corneal aberrations and internal optical aberrations, particularly those of the crystalline lens. Therefore, to measure the eye's total aberrations prior to a corneal laser procedure, a wavefront sensing device—not corneal topography—should be used (Artal et al, 2001).

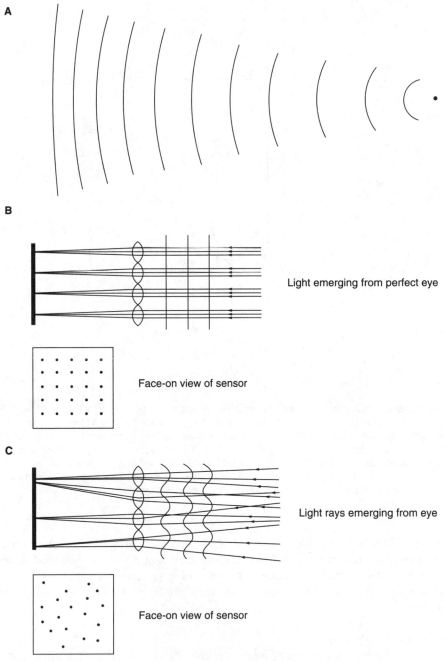

FIGURE 15-14A. As the distance from an object increases, the wavefronts become flatter. When the object is located at infinity, the wavefronts are flat. **B.** Flat wavefronts cause a regular grid pattern to be formed on the sensor of the Hartmann-Shack aberrometer. **C.** The aberrations of the eye cause the wavefronts that emerge from the eye to be distorted. These distorted wavefronts result in an irregular grid pattern.

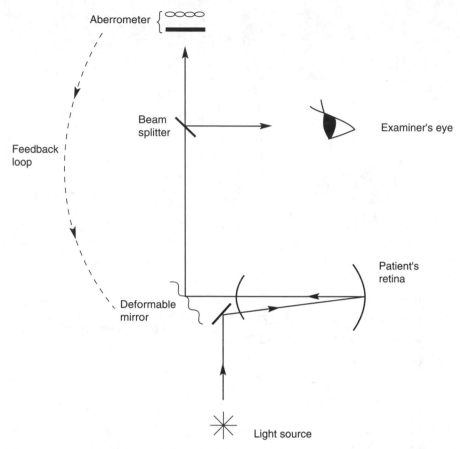

FIGURE 15-15. Instruments that incorporate adaptive optics can be used to obtain high-resolution images of ocular structures. Light is reflected off a plane mirror into the eye, illuminating the retina. This light is subsequently reflected off the retina and onto a deformable mirror that, in turn, reflects the light through a beam splitter and onto the Hartmann-Shack aberrometer. The aberrometer provides feedback to the deformable mirror, and this feedback is used to adjust the deformable mirror such that aberrations are minimized. An examiner obtains a high-resolution view of the retina when the aberrations are minimized. (This schematic diagram is a simplification.)

stability of these corrections depends on the physical properties of the cornea. The cornea is not a stable, uniform material such as a piece of plastic or glass— it is a living tissue that is not uniform in its composition. Consequently, the stable, long-term correction of aberrations through corneal shaping will be challenging.

Imaging the Fundus

Adaptive optics has important implications for viewing the fundus. When the fundus is viewed with an ophthalmosope, the clarity of the image seen by the clinician is limited by the same aberrations that limit the patient's vision. If we could compensate for the optical aberrations, the fundus could be seen in greater detail (Liang et al., 1997). Adaptive optics allows for this compensation, and retinal imaging devices that include adaptive optics are likely to prove invaluable for patient care (Fig. 15-15).

CHROMATIC ABERRATIONS

Seidel aberrations are present with monochromatic light. In comparison, chromatic aberrations are present only when the light is a mixture of wavelengths—when the light is *polychromatic*. Chromatic aberrations occur because the speed of light in a refractive medium varies with the wavelength of light. When light enters a denser refractive medium, the speed of short-wavelength light is more retarded than the speed of longer-wavelength light.

Figure 15-16 shows white light—a combination of light of different wavelengths—incident upon a prism. The emergent light forms a spectrum of colors.[12] The shorter wavelengths (higher index of refraction) are refracted to a greater extent than are the longer wavelengths. This separation of white light into its component elements by a prism (or other optical element) is referred to as *dispersion*.

Just as prisms disperse light, so do lenses. In Figure 15-17, white light is incident upon a plus lens. Since the index of refraction is higher for the shorter wavelengths, they are focused closer to the lens. The distance between the focal point of the wavelength that is most refracted (which results in the perception of blue or violet) and the wavelength that is least refracted (which results in the

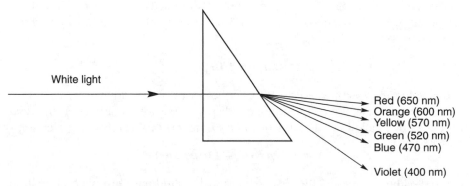

FIGURE 15-16. White light, incident upon a prism, forms a spectrum of colors because the index of refraction varies with wavelength, with the index of refraction being greatest for short wavelengths. One nanometer (nm) is equal to 10^{-9}m.

---

[12] The color of light is dependent on its wavelength. Wavelength is a physical property, and color is a perception.

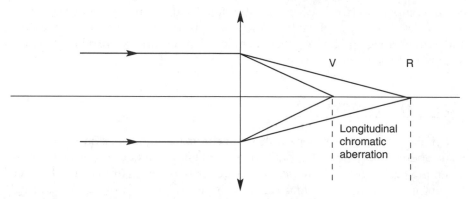

FIGURE 15-17. Longitudinal chromatic aberration is the distance between the visible wavelength that is most refracted (represented by the color violet) and the visible wavelength that is least refracted (represented by the color red).

perception of red) is a measure of the *longitudinal chromatic aberration* of the lens.

Dispersive Power and Constrigence

In most cases, a single index of refraction is specified for a given refractive medium. For instance, the index of refraction for crown glass is typically specified as 1.52. This value is the index of refraction for a specific wavelength: 589 nm. As we have just learned, the index of refraction is different for other wavelengths.

To quantify the amount of dispersion produced by a prism or lens, we use three wavelengths: 486, 589, and 656 nm. The indices of refraction for these wavelengths are designated as n_c, n_d, and n_f, respectively.[13] The *dipersive power* (ω) is given by

$$\omega = (n_f - n_c)/(n_d - 1)$$

As this value increases, the dispersion of the prism or lens increases.

As given below, the reciprocal of the dispersive power is defined as the *constrigence* (also called the *V-value* or *Abbe's number*) of the refracting element:

$$V = 1 / \omega = (n_d - 1)/(n_f - n_c)$$

As the *V*-value increases, the dispersion and longitudinal chromatic aberration decrease.

---

[13] These wavelengths are absent in the sunlight that reaches the earth, creating dark lines in the solar spectrum that are called *Fraunhofer lines.*

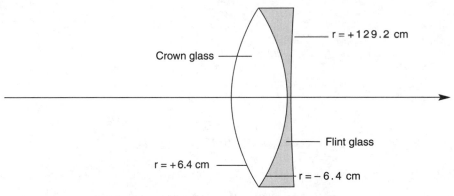

FIGURE 15-18. An achromatic doublet formed by cementing a biconvex crown glass lens to a minus flint glass lens. Radii of curvature are given for the surfaces. See text for further details.

Achromatic Lenses

To minimize longitudinal chromatic aberrations, we can combine a lens of a given index of refraction with a lens of another index of refraction to form an *achromatic doublet*. The component lenses of the doublet are in contact with each other. One of the lenses has a positive refractive power and the other a negative refractive power (Fig.15-18). The formulae used to calculate the powers of the component lenses are given below:

$$P_1/V_1 = -P_2/V_2$$
$$P_t = P_1 + P_2$$

where

P_1 = the power of the first lens in air
P_2 = the power of the second lens in air
V_1 = the constrigence for the first lens
V_2 = the constrigence for the second lens
P_t = the total power of the achromatic doublet

Let us apply these formulae. *Using a plus crown glass lens with a constrigence of 59.0 and a minus flint glass lens (n = 1.62) with a constrigence of 37.0, design a +6.00 D achromatic doublet that minimizes longitudinal chromatic aberration. Specifically, what are the powers of the component lenses?*

$$P_1/V_1 = -P_2/V_2$$
$$P_1/59 = -P_2/37$$

and

$$P_t = P_1 + P_2$$

$$+6.00 \text{ D} = P_1 + P_2$$

Thus

$$P_1 = -1.59 P_2$$

Therefore

$$+6.00D = -1.59 P_2 + P_2$$
$$P_2 = -10.17 \text{ D}$$

and

$$+6.00 \text{ D} = P_1 + -10.17 \text{ D}$$
$$P_1 = +16.17 \text{ D}$$

These calculations tell us that the power of the crown glass lens in air is +16.17 D and the power of the flint glass lens in air is –10.17 D. To create an achromatic doublet with a combined power of +6.00 D, these two lenses are cemented together (Fig. 15-18).

Assume that the plus crown glass lens is equiconvex. What are the radii of curvature of the four lens surfaces? Since the radii of curvature (absolute values) for the front and back surfaces of the crown glass lens are equal, the powers of the two surfaces must also be equal. For the front surface, we have

$$P = (n' - n)/r$$
$$+8.08 \text{ D} = (1.52 - 1.00)/r$$
$$r = +0.064 \text{ m or } +6.4 \text{ cm}$$

The radius of curvature for the front surface of this equiconvex lens is +6.4 cm and for the back surface, –6.4 cm. From Figure 15-18, we see that the front surface of the flint glass lens has the same curvature as the back surface of the crown glass lens. The power of the front surface of the flint glass lens in air is

$$P = (n' - n)/r$$
$$P = (1.62 - 1.00)/-0.064 \text{ m}$$
$$P = -9.69 \text{ D}$$

Since the total power of the flint glass lens is –10.17 D, the power of its back surface is –0.48 D. Its radius of curvature is

$$P = (n' - n)/r$$
$$-0.48 \text{ D} = (1.00 - 1.62)/r$$
$$r = +1.29 \text{ m or } +129.2 \text{ cm}$$

The radii of curvature of all four surfaces of the +6.00 D achromatic doublet are given in Figure 15-18.

Although the calculations give the powers of the lenses in air, the components of the doublet are fused to each other. To convince ourselves that the fused doublet has a total power of +6.00 D, let us add together the powers of the three interfaces. For the first interface (air/crown glass) the power is +8.08 D; for the third interface (flint glass/air), the power is –0.48 D. To complete this calculation, we must determine the power at the crown glass/flint glass interface, as follows:

$$P = (n' - n)/r$$
$$P = (1.62 - 1.52)/-0.064 \text{ m}$$
$$P = -1.56 \text{ D}$$

Adding together the powers of the three interfaces, we obtain a total power of approximately +6.00 D.

CHROMATIC ABERRATIONS OF THE HUMAN EYE

The human eye exhibits about 0.75 D of longitudinal chromatic aberration (Kruger et al., 1993). This corresponds to a linear distance of 0.25 mm. We are not normally aware of this longitudinal chromatic aberration.

Longitudinal chromatic aberration is thought to be a stimulus to accommodation. In Figure 15-19A, an eye is focused on point *B*. The image of point *A* (i.e., *A'*) is anterior to the retina and produces the same amount of retinal blur

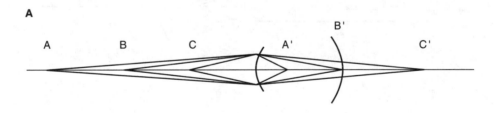

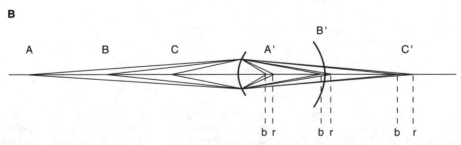

FIGURE 15-19A. Points *A, B,* and *C* result in the images *A', B',* and *C'.* **B.** Upon closer inspection, we see that each of the images (*A', B',* and *C'*) suffers from longitudinal chromatic aberration. For the image *C',* blue (*b*) is focused closer to the retina, and for the image *A',* red (*r*) is focused closer to the retina. The visual system may use this information to determine if accommodation should be increased (as is required to focus on *C*) or decreased (as is required to focus on *A*).

as the image of point C (i.e., C'), which is posterior to the retina. Suppose the subject wishes to change his or her fixation to point A. Since this point's image (A') has the same amount of retinal blur as C', how does the accommodative system know if it should increase or decrease its power?

Figure 15-19B shows the longitudinal chromatic aberration present in the images A', B', and C'. For C', the shorter wavelengths are focused closer to the retina than the longer wavelengths. For A', the longer wavelengths are focused closer to the retina. If the accommodative system were able to use this information, it could accommodate in the correct direction (i.e., increase its power for the near object and decrease its power for the far object). Recent research suggests that chromatic aberration is indeed a cue to accommodation. For instance, the ability to accommodate accurately is impaired under monochromatic conditions (Aggarwala et al., 1995).

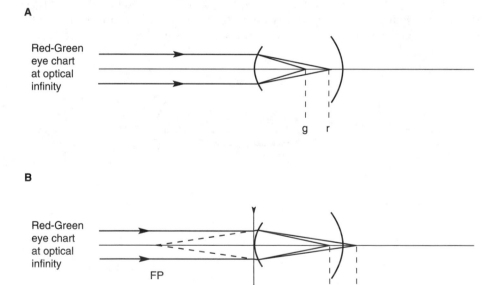

FIGURE 15-20A. When a patient views a red-green acuity chart, green images (*g*) are focused in front of the red images (*r*). In a myopic eye (or an emmetropic eye viewing through a plus lens), the optotypes on both the red and green backgrounds are focused in front of the retina. **B.** The goal of the red-green refraction technique is to straddle the retina with the green and red images such that they are positioned equally distant from the retina and appear equally clear to the patient. This occurs when the appropriate correction—in this case a minus lens to correct the myopia—is in place.

THE RED-GREEN REFRACTION TECHNIQUE[14]

This commonly used refraction procedure takes advantage of the eye's longitudinal chromatic aberration. When a patient views a projected visual acuity chart that is green on one side and red on the other side, the green image is focused anterior to the red image. If the patient is myopic, both the green and red images are focused anterior to the retina and both will appear blurred (Fig. 15-20A). However, the optotypes on the red background appear less blurred because they are focused closer to the retina than the optotypes on the green background.

When the duochrome test is performed in the clinic, plus lenses may be placed in front of the patient's eye so that both the green and red images fall anterior to the retina.[15] Under these conditions, the optotypes on the red background appear clearer than those on the green background. The amount of minus power is then increased in a stepwise fashion (0.25 or 0.50 D per step) until the letters on the green background are just slightly clearer than those on the red background. The lens power is subsequently adjusted, so that the letters on the green background and those on the red background are equally clear (Fig. 15–20B). When this occurs, the green and red images straddle the retina, with each the same distance (dioptrically) from the retina.

LATERAL (TRANSVERSE) CHROMATIC ABERRATION

Figure 15-21A shows a lens that has no longitudinal aberration. However, the image still suffers from *lateral chromatic aberration*: each wavelength results in an image of a different size. Consequently, the image has colored fringes.

Lateral chromatic aberration can be minimized with an optical system consisting of two lenses of the same constringence that are separated by the distance *d,* as defined below:

$$d = (f_1' + f_2') / 2$$

Figure 15-21B shows a lens system with minimal lateral chromatic aberration. Note, however, that the amount of longitudinal aberration is substantial. Depending on the intended use of an optical system, it may be a priority either to minimize longitudinal chromatic aberration or to minimize lateral chromatic aberration.

---

[14] This is also called the *duochrome* or *bichrome* refractive technique.

[15] Since the images for an uncorrected myope fall anterior to the retina, it is not necessary to add plus lenses. For an emmetrope or hyperope, however, plus lenses must be placed in front of the eye so that the images are focused anterior to the retina.

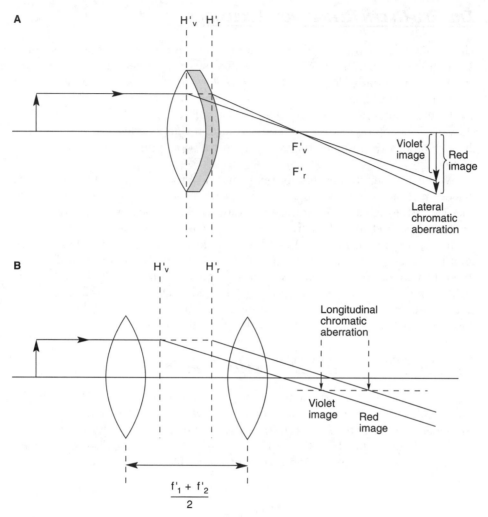

FIGURE 15-21A. Each wavelength has a different principal plane. A lens has no longitudinal chromatic aberration when the principal planes (H'_v and H'_r) are separated such that the focal points for shortest and longest wavelengths are coincident. When this occurs, however, there is substantial lateral chromatic aberration. **B.** When two lenses are separated by an appropriate distance, lateral chromatic aberration is eliminated. Under these conditions, however, there is substantial longitudinal aberration.

BIBLIOGRAPHY

Aggarwala KR, Nowbotsing S, Kruber PB. Accommodation to monochromatic and white-light targets. *Invest Vis Sci* 1995;13:2595.

Applegate RA. Limits to vision: can we do better than nature? *J Refract Surgy* 2000;16:S547.

Artel P, Guirao A, Berrio E, Williams DR. Compensation of corneal aberrations by internal optics of the human eye. *J Vis* 2001;1:1.

Guirao A, Redondo M, Artal P. Optical aberrations of the human eye as a function of age. *J Opt Soc Am A* 2000;17:1697.

Ivanoff A. About the spherical aberration of the eye. *J Opt Soc Am* 1956;46:901.

Kruger PB, Mathews S, Aggarwala KR, Sanchez N. Chromatic aberration and ocular focus: Fincham revisited. *Vis Res* 1993;33:1397.

Liang J, Grimm B, Goetz S, Bille JF. Objective measurement of wave aberrations of the human eye with the use of a Hartmann-Shack wave-front sensor. *J Opt Soc Am A* 994;11:1949.

Liang J, Williams DR. Aberrations and retinal image quality of the normal human eye. *J Opt Soc Am A* 1997;14:2873.

Liang J, Williams DR, Miller DT. Supernormal vision and high-resolution retinal imaging through adaptive optics. *J Opt Soc Am A* 1997;14:2884.

Thibos LN. Principles of Hartmann-Shack aberrometry. *J Refract Surg* 2000;16:S563.

Self-Assessment Problems

1. An emmetropic subject, whose pupil has been pharmacologically dilated, views a distant point source through an opaque disk that has two small holes (each hole is about 1 mm in diameter) drilled through it.[16] The two holes are separated by about 8 mm. (a) Will the patient see a single point source or two points? Why? (b) What happens when the subject places her finger in front of the top hole? Explain.

2. Do you expect the amount of positive spherical aberration in a myopic eye to increase or decrease following a standard LASIK procedure? Why?

3. (a) Does a rigid spherical contact lens neutralize the eye's Siedel aberrations? Explain your anwer. (b) Is it theoretically possible to correct the eye's Siedel aberrations with a contact lens?

4. (a) Determine the bending factor for a +5.00 DS equiconvex plastic lens. (b) What is the shape of a +5.00 DS lens that has minimal spherical aberration? (c) When worn by a patient, which surface of the lens should face the patient's eye?

5. An achromatic doublet is to be constructed from the materials listed below:

	n_c	n_d	n_f
Glass 1	1.57	1.59	1.61
Glass 2	1.70	1.73	1.76

(a) To construct a +10.00 DS achromatic doublet, what should be the powers of the component lenses? (b) Assume that the lens made of glass 1 is biconvex. What are the radii of curvature of the four lens surfaces?

6. Determine the dispersive power of glass 1 in Problem 5.

7. An optical system consists of +7.00 DS and +4.00 DS lenses. To minimize lateral chromatic aberration, what should the separation of the lenses be?

---

[16] This disk is referred to as a *Scheiner* disk.

Answers to Self-Assessment Problems

1. $n \sin \theta = n' \sin \theta'$
$(1.33) \sin \theta = (1.00) \sin 45°$
$\theta = 32.1°$

2. $n \sin \theta = n' \sin \theta'$
$(1.00) \sin 25° = (1.33) \sin \theta'$
$\theta' = 18.53°$

If the ray was not deviated:

Tan $25° = d/200.00$ cm
$d = 93.26$ cm

But because the ray is refracted:

Tan $18.53° = d/200.00$ cm
$d = 67.04$ cm

Therefore the deviation of the ray is

93.26 cm $- 67.04$ cm $= 26.22$ cm

3. At the first interface:

$n \sin \theta = n' \sin \theta'$
$(1.00) \sin 30° = 1.52 \sin \theta'$
$\theta' = 19.2°$

A ─────────────────────────────

At the second interface:

$$n \sin \theta = n' \sin \theta'$$
$$(1.52) \sin 19.52° = (1.00) \sin \theta'$$
$$\theta' = 30.0°$$

4. $$n \sin \theta = n' \sin \theta'$$
$$(1.72) \sin \theta = (1.00) \sin 90°$$
$$\theta = 35.5°$$

5. $$n \sin \theta = n' \sin \theta'$$
$$(2.42) \sin \theta = (1.33) \sin 90°$$
$$\theta = 33.3°$$

CHAPTER 2.
REFRACTION AT SPHERICAL SURFACES

1. A. Positive

   B. $| P | = | (n' - n)/r |$
   $| P | = |(1.52 - 1.00)/0.15 \text{ m}|$
   $P = +3.47 \text{ D}$

   C. $| P | = | n/f |$
   $| 3.47 \text{ D} | = | (1.00)(100)/f |$
   $| f | = | 28.82 \text{ cm} |$
   $| P | = | n'/f' |$
   $| 3.47 \text{ D} | = | (1.52)(100)/f' |$
   $| f' | = | 43.80 \text{ cm} |$

   F is 28.82 cm to the left of the surface, and F' is 43.80 cm to the right of the surface.

2. A. Negative.

   B. $| P | = | (n' - n)/r |$
   $| P | = | (1.52 - 1.00)/0.20 \text{ m} |$
   $P = -2.60 \text{ D}$

   C. $| P | = | n/f |$

$$| \; 2.60 \; D \; | \; = \; | \; (1.00)(100)/f \; |$$
$$| \; f \; | \; = \; | \; 38.46 cm \; |$$
$$| \; P \; | \; = \; | \; n'/f' \; |$$
$$| \; 2.60 \; D \; | \; = \; | \; (1.52)(100)/f' \; |$$
$$| \; f' \; | \; = \; | \; 58.46 \; cm \; |$$

F is located 38.46 cm to the right of the surface, and F' is located 58.46 cm to the left of the surface.

3. A. Positive.

B. Negative.

C. Positive.

D. Negative.

4. A.
$$| \; P \; | \; = \; | \; n/f \; |$$
$$| \; {-}10.00 \; D \; | \; = \; | \; (1.00)(100)/f \; |$$
$$| \; f \; | \; = \; | \; 10.00 \; cm \; |$$

F is 10.00 cm to the right of the diverging surface.

$$| \; P \; | \; = \; | \; n'/f' \; |$$
$$| \; {-}10.00 \; D \; | \; = \; | \; (1.52)(100)/f' \; |$$
$$| \; f' \; | \; = \; | \; 15.2 \; cm \; |$$

F' is 15.2 cm to the left of the diverging surface.

B. The image distance is about 7.2 cm to the left of the surface. The image height is about 1.4 cm.

C. The magnification is $| \; 1.4 \; cm/3.0 \; cm \; | \; = \; | \; 0.5X \; |$
Since the image is erect, the magnification is designated as +0.5X.

D. The image is erect. Because it is formed by diverging light rays, the image is virtual. The image can be seen, but can not be focused on a screen.

5. A.
$$| \; P \; | \; = \; | \; n/f \; |$$
$$| \; {+}10.00 \; D \; | \; = \; | \; 1.00/f \; |$$
$$| \; f \; | \; = \; | \; 10.00 \; cm \; |$$

F is 10.00 cm to the left of the converging surface.

$$| \; P \; | \; = \; | \; n'/f' \; |$$
$$| \; {+}10.00 D \; | \; = \; | \; 1.52/f' \; |$$
$$| \; f' \; | \; = \; | \; 15.2 \; cm \; |$$

F' is 15.2 cm to the right of the converging surface.

B. Image distance is 30.4 cm to the right of the surface. The image height is 2.0 cm.

C. The magnification is $|2.0 \text{ cm}/2.0 \text{ cm}| = |1.0X|$
Because the image is inverted, the magnification is $-1.0X$

D. The image is inverted. Because it is formed by converging light rays that could be focused onto a screen, it is real.

6. A. The image appears closer to the surface.

B. The diverging light rays that are emitted by the rock are further diverged at the surface of the pond (at the water–air interface). The rays appear to come from a point that is less than 3.0 m from the surface. Because the image is formed by diverging light rays, it is virtual (see Fig. 3-7).

CHAPTER 3.
THE VERGENCE RELATIONSHIP

1. A. $\quad\quad P = (n' - n)/r$
$-10.00 \text{ D} = (1.52 - 1.00)/r$
$r = -0.052 \text{ m or } -5.2 \text{ cm}$

B. $\quad\quad P = n'/f'$
$-10.00D = 1.52/f'$
$f' = -0.152 \text{ m or } -15.2 \text{ cm}$

C. $\quad\quad P = -n/f$
$-10.00 \text{ D} = -1.00/f$
$f = +0.100 \text{ m or } +10.0 \text{ cm}$

2. A. $\quad\quad P = (n' - n)/r$
$+20.00D = (1.50 - 1.00)/r$
$r = + 0.025 \text{ m or } +2.5 \text{ cm}$

B. $\quad\quad P = n'/f'$
$+20.00 \text{ D} = 1.50/f'$
$f' = +0.075 \text{ m or } +7.5 \text{ cm}$

A

C.
$$P = -n/f$$
$$+20.00 \text{ D} = -1.00/f$$
$$f = -0.050 \text{ m or } -5.0 \text{ cm}$$

3. A.
$$P = (n' - n)/r$$
$$P = (1.52 - 1.00)/+0.15 \text{ m}$$
$$P = +3.47 \text{ D}$$

B.
$$P = n'/f'$$
$$+3.47D = 1.52 / f'$$
$$f' = +0.438 \text{ m or } +43.8 \text{ cm}$$

C.
$$P = n/f$$
$$+3.47D = -1.00/f$$
$$f = -0.288 \text{ m or } -28.8 \text{ cm}$$

4.
$$P = (n' - n)/r$$
$$P = (1.58 - 1.00)/-0.125 \text{ m}$$
$$P = -4.64 \text{ D}$$

5. A.
$$L' = L + P$$
$$L' = (1.00/-0.20 \text{ m}) + (-10.00 \text{ D})$$
$$L' = -15.00 \text{ D}$$
$$L' = n'/l'$$
$$-15.00 \text{ D} = 1.52/l'$$
$$l' = -0.101 m \text{ or } -10.1 cm$$
$$M = L/L'$$
$$M = -5.00 \text{ D}/-15.00 \text{ D}$$
$$M = +0.33X$$
$$(6.00 \text{ mm})(+0.33X) = +2.00 \text{ mm}$$

B. Virtual.

C. Erect.

6. A.
$$L' = L + P$$
$$L' = (1.00/-0.20 \text{ m}) + (+10.00 \text{ D})$$
$$L' = +5.00 \text{ D}$$
$$L' = n'/l'$$
$$+5.00D = 1.52/l'$$
$$l' = +0.304 \text{ m or } +30.4 \text{ cm}$$
$$M = L/L'$$

$$M = -5.00 \text{ D}/+5.00 \text{ D}$$
$$M = -1.00X$$
$$(10.00 \text{ mm})(-1.00X) = -10.00 \text{ mm}$$

B. Real.

C. Inverted.

7. A.
$$L' = L + P$$
$$L' = (1.00/-0.050 \text{ m}) + (+10.00 \text{ D})$$
$$L' = -10.00 \text{ D}$$
$$L' = n'/l'$$
$$-10.00 \text{ D} = 1.52/l'$$
$$l' = -0.152 \text{ m or } -15.2 \text{ cm}$$
$$M = L/L'$$
$$M = -20.00 \text{ D}/-10.00 \text{ D}$$
$$M = +2.00X$$
$$(10.00 \text{ mm})(+2.00X) = +20.00 \text{ mm}$$

B. Virtual.

C. Erect.

8.
$$L' = L + P$$
$$1.52/-0.05 \text{ m} = L + 15.00 \text{ D}$$
$$L = -45.40 \text{ D}$$
$$L = n/l$$
$$-45.40 \text{ D} = 1.00/l$$
$$l = -0.022 \text{ m or } -2.2 \text{ cm}$$

9.
$$L' = L + P$$
$$1.52/+0.20 \text{ m} = L + 15.00 \text{ D}$$
$$L = -7.40 \text{ D}$$
$$L = n/l$$
$$-7.40 \text{ D} = 1.00/l$$
$$l = -0.135 \text{ m or } -13.5 \text{ cm}$$

10.
$$L' = L + P$$
$$L' = 1.33/-3.00 \text{ m} + 0.00 \text{ D}$$
$$L' = -0.44 \text{ D}$$
$$L' = n'/l'$$
$$-0.44D = 1.00/l'$$
$$l' = -2.27 \text{ m}$$

A

The virtual image of the rock is located 2.27 m below the surface of the pond. Consequently, the rock appears to be 2.27 m below the surface of the pond.

11. This problem can be confusing because it is easy to incorrectly use the linear sign convention. For instance, if you draw a diagram that shows the pupil to the right of the cornea, you must assume that light travels from right to left; this is not consistent with our linear sign convention. Alternatively, you could draw the diagram with the pupil to the left of the cornea and then use the linear sign convention. This is the approach we will take to solve this problem.

The first step is to determine the power of the cornea. We treat the cornea as a spherical refracting surface that separates the aqueous from water. The cornea is assumed to have no thickness and no index of refraction. It simply gives shape to the aqueous-air interface. Its power is as follows:

$$P = (n' - n)/r$$
$$P = (1.000 - 1.333)/)/-0.0078 \text{ m}$$
$$P = +42.69 \text{ D}$$

The object (the pupil) is located in the aqueous and is 3.60 mm from the cornea:

$$L' = L + P$$
$$L' = [(1.333)(1000)/-3.60 \text{ mm}] + 42.69 \text{ D}$$
$$L' = -327.59 \text{ D}$$
$$L' = n'/l'$$
$$-327.59 \text{ D} = (1.000)(1000)/l'$$
$$l' = -3.05 \text{ mm}$$

When you look into someone's eye, you see a virtual image of the pupil that is located nearer to the cornea (3.05 mm) than the actual pupil (3.60 mm).

12.
$$M = L/L'$$
$$M = -370.28 \text{ D}/-327.59 \text{ D}$$
$$M = +1.13X$$
$$(4.00 \text{ mm})(+1.13X) = +4.52 \text{ mm}$$

The (virtual) image of the pupil that you see when looking into the eye is larger than the actual pupil.

A ━━━━━━━━━━━━━━━━━━━━━━━━━━━━━━

1. A. $P_1 = (n' - n)/r$
$P_1 = (1.52 - 1.00)/+0.08$
$P_1 = +6.50$ D
$P_2 = (n' - n)/r$
$P_2 = (1.00 - 1.52)/-0.06$ m
$P_2 = +8.67$ D

For a thin lens:

$P_T = P_1 + P_2$
$P_T = +6.50$ D $+ 8.67$ D
$P_T = +15.17$ D

B. $P = 1.00/f'$
15.17 D $= (1.00)(100)/f'$
$f' = +6.59$ cm

The secondary focal point is located 6.59 cm to the right of the lens. Since the primary focal length of a thin lens is equal to the secondary focal length (in absolute values), the primary focal point is 6.59 cm to the left of the lens.

2. A. $L' = L + P$
$L' = [(1.00)(100)/-15.00$ cm$] + 20.00$ D
$L' = +13.33$ D
$L' = n'/l'$
$+13.33$ D $= (1.00)(100)/l'$
$l' = +7.50$ cm
$M = L/L'$
$M = -6.67$ D$/+13.33$ D
$M = -0.50X$

Since the index of refraction is the same on both sides of the thin lens, magnification can also be calculated as

$M = l'/l$
$M = +7.50$ cm$/-15.00$ cm
$M = -0.50X$
$(13.00$ mm$)$ $(0.50X) = -6.50$ mm

A

B. Real because it is formed by converging light.

C. Inverted.

3. A.

$$L' = L + P$$
$$L' = [(1.00)(100)/-5.00 \text{ cm}] + 10.00 \text{ D}$$
$$L' = -10.00 \text{ D}$$
$$L' = n'/l'$$
$$-10.00 \text{ D} = (1.00)(100)/l'$$
$$l' = -10.00 \text{ cm}$$
$$M = L/L'$$
$$M = -20.00 \text{ D}/-10.00 \text{ D}$$
$$M = +2.00X$$
$$(30.00 \text{ mm})(+2.00X) = +60.00 \text{ mm}$$

B. Virtual, because it is formed by diverging light.

C. Erect.

4. A.

$$L' = L + P$$
$$L' = (1.00)(100)/-10.00 \text{ cm} + (-30.00 \text{ D})$$
$$L' = -40.00 \text{ D}$$
$$L' = n'/l'$$
$$-40.00 \text{ D} = (1.00)(100)/l'$$
$$l' = -2.50 \text{ cm}$$
$$M = L/L'$$
$$M = -10.00 \text{ D}/-40.00 \text{ D}$$
$$M = +0.25X$$
$$(30.00 \text{ mm})(+0.25X) = +7.50 \text{ mm}$$

B. Virtual.

C. Erect.

5.

$$L' = L + P$$
$$(1.00)(100)/+50.00 \text{ cm} = L + (+25.00 \text{ D})$$
$$L = -23.00 \text{ D}$$
$$L = n/l$$
$$-23.00 \text{ D} = (1.00)(100)/l$$
$$l = -4.35 \text{ cm}$$

When an object is located 4.35 cm to the left of this plus lens, a real image is focused 50.00 cm to the right of the lens.

6. $L' = L + P$

$(1.00)(100)/-50.00 \text{ cm} = L + (+25.00 \text{ D})$

$$L = -27.00 \text{ D}$$
$$L = n/l$$
$$-27.00 \text{ D} = (1.00)(100)/l$$
$$l = -3.70 \text{ cm}$$

When an object is located 3.70 cm to the left of this plus lens, a virtual image is formed 50.00 cm to the left of the lens. Since the object is located within the focal length of this thin plus lens, the image is virtual and magnified.

7.

$$L' = L + P$$
$(1.00)(100)/-10.00 \text{ cm} = L + (-5.00 \text{ D})$
$$L = -5.00 \text{ D}$$
$$L = n/l$$
$$-5.00 \text{ D} = (1.00)(100)/l$$
$$l = -20.00 \text{cm}$$

When an object is located 20.00 cm to the left of this negative lens, a virtual image is formed 10.00 cm to the left of the lens.

8.

$$(x)(x') = f^2$$
$$(0.25 \text{ m})(0.40 \text{ m}) = f^2$$
$$f = 0.32 \text{ m}$$
$$P = n/f'$$
$$P = 1.00/+0.32 \text{ m}$$
$$P = +3.13 \text{ D}$$

CHAPTER 5.
OPTICAL SYSTEMS WITH MULTIPLE SURFACES

1. A. <u>Power of first surface:</u>

$P_1 = (n' - n) / r$

$P_1 = (1.52 - 1.00) / +0.05 \text{ m}$

$P_1 = +10.40 \text{ D}$

Power of the second surface:

$P_2 = (n' - n) / r$

$P_2 = (1.00 - 1.52) / -0.025$ m

$P_2 = +20.80$ D

Refraction at first surface:

$L' = L + P$

$L' = [(1.00)(100) / -25.00$ cm] + 10.40 D

$L' = -4.00$ D + 10.40 D

$L' = +6.40$D

$L' = n' / l'$

+6.40 D = $(1.52)(100) / l'$

$l' = +23.75$ cm

This real image is located 23.75 cm to the right of the first surface and 20.75 cm to the right of the second surface (i.e., 23.75 cm −3.00 cm = 20.75 cm). It serves as a virtual object for the second surface. Keep in mind that the rays that form this virtual object exist in the glass.

Refraction at second surface:

$L' = L + P$

$L' = [(1.52)(100) / +20.75$ cm] + 20.80 D

$L' = +7.33$D + 20.80 D

$L' = +28.13$ D

The light rays that form this real image exist in air.

$L' = n' / l'$

+28.13 D = $(1.00)(100) / l'$

$l' = +3.55$ cm

The image is located 3.55 cm to the right of the second lens surface.

B. $M_T = (M_1)(M_2)$

$M_T = (-4.00 \text{ D}/ +6.40 \text{ D}) / (+7.33 \text{ D} / +28.13 \text{ D})$

$M_T = -0.16X$

$(30.00 \text{ mm})(-0.16X) = -4.80 \text{ mm}$

C.   Since the final image is formed by converging light rays, it is real.

D.   The final real image is inverted. This is indicated by the negative sign that is given for the total magnification.

2. A.   <u>Power of first surface:</u>

$P_1 = (n' - n) / r$

$P_1 = (1.52 - 1.00) / +0.12 \text{ m}$

$P_1 = +4.33 \text{ D}$

<u>Power of the second surface:</u>

$P_2 = (n' - n) / r$

$P_2 = (1.00 - 1.52) / -0.07 \text{ m}$

$P_2 = +7.43 \text{ D}$

<u>Refraction at first surface:</u>

$L' = L + P$

$L' = [(1.00)(100) / -3.00 \text{ cm}] + 4.33 \text{ D}$

$L' = -33.33 \text{ D} + 4.33 \text{ D}$

$L' = -29.00 \text{ D}$

$L' = n' / l'$

$-29.00 \text{D} = (1.52)(100) / l'$

$l' = -5.24 \text{ cm}$

This virtual image is located 5.24 cm to the left of the first surface and 7.74 cm (i.e., 5.24 cm +2.50 cm = 7.74 cm) to the left of the second surface. The rays that form this image exist in glass. It serves as the object for the second surface.

Refraction at second surface:

$L' = L + P$

$L' = [(1.52)(100) / -7.74 \text{ cm}] + 7.43 \text{ D}$

$L' = -19.64 \text{ D} + 7.43 \text{ D}$

$L' = -12.21 \text{ D}$

The light rays that form this virtual image exist in air.

$L' = n' / l'$

$-12.21 \text{ D} = (1.00)(100) / l'$

$l' = -8.19 \text{ cm}$

The image is located 8.19 cm to the left of the second lens surface.

B. $M_T = (M_1)(M_2)$

$M_T = (-33.33 \text{ D} / -29.00 \text{ D}) / (-19.64 \text{ D} / -12.21 \text{ D})$

$M_T = +1.85X$

$(30.00 \text{ mm})(+1.85X) = +55.5 \text{ mm}$

C. The final image is formed by diverging light rays—it is to the left of the second surface. Therefore the final image is virtual.

D. This virtual image is erect as indicated by the plus sign for magnification.

3. A. Power of first surface:

$P_1 = (n' - n) / r$

$P_1 = (1.52 - 1.00) / +0.15 \text{ m}$

$P_1 = +3.47 \text{ D}$

Power of the second surface:

$P_2 = (n' - n) / r$

$P_2 = (1.00 - 1.52) / +0.15 \text{ m}$

$P_2 = -3.47 \text{ D}$

Refraction at first surface:

$L' = L + P$

$L' = [(1.00)(100) / -40.00 \text{ cm}] + (+3.47 \text{ D})$

$L' = -2.50 \text{ D} + (+3.47 \text{ D})$

$L' = +0.97 \text{ D}$

$L' = n' / l'$

$+0.97 \text{ D} = (1.52)(100) / l'$

$l' = +156.70 \text{ cm}$

This real image is located 156.70 cm to the right of the first surface and 153.70 cm (i.e., 156.70 cm −3.00 cm = 153.70 cm) to the right of the second surface. It serves as a virtual object for the second surface. Keep in mind that the rays that form this virtual object exist in the glass.

Refraction at second surface:

$L' = L + P$

$L' = [(1.52)(100) / +153.70 \text{ cm}] + (-3.47 \text{ D})$

$L' = +0.99 \text{ D} + (-3.47 \text{ D})$

$L' = -2.48 \text{ D}$

The rays that form this virtual image exist in air.

$L' = n' / l'$

$-2.48 \text{ D} = (1.00)(100) / l'$

$l' = -40.32 \text{ cm}$

The image is located 40.32 cm to the left of the second lens surface.

A

B. $M_T = (M_1)(M_2)$

   $M_T = (-2.50 \text{ D} / +0.97 \text{ D}) / (+0.99 \text{ D} / -2.48 \text{ D})$

   $M_T = +1.03X$

   $(30.00 \text{ mm})(+1.03X) = +30.90 \text{ mm}$

C.   Since the final image is formed by diverging light rays, it is virtual.

D.   The final virtual image is erect as indicated by the positive sign of the magnification.

4. A.   <u>Refraction at first lens</u>:

   $L' = L + P$

   $L' = [(1.00)(100) / -30.00 \text{ cm}] + (-10.00 \text{ D})$

   $L' = -3.33 \text{ D} + (-10.00 \text{ D})$

   $L\varpi = -13.33 \text{ D}$

   $L' = n' / l'$

   $-13.33 \text{ D} = (1.00)(100) / l'$

   $l' = -7.50 \text{ cm}$

This virtual image is located 7.50 cm to the left of the first lens and 10.00 cm (i.e., 7.50 cm + 2.50 cm = 10.00 cm) to the left of the second lens. Keep in mind that the rays that form this image exist in *air*. It serves as an object for the second lens.

   <u>Refraction at second lens</u>:

   $L' = L + P$

   $L' = [(1.00)(100) / -10.00 \text{ cm}] + (+1.00 \text{ D})$

   $L' = -10.00 \text{ D} + (+1.00 \text{ D})$

   $L' = -9.00 \text{ D}$

   $L' = n' / l'$

   $-9.00 \text{ D} = (1.00)(100) / l'$

$l' = -11.11$ cm

The virtual image is located 11.11 cm to the left of the second lens.

B.　$M_T = (M_1)(M_2)$

　　$M_T = (-3.33$ D $/ -13.33$ D$) / (-10.00$ D $/ -9.00$ D$)$

　　$M_T = +0.28X$

　　$(45.00$ mm$)(+0.28X) = +12.60$ mm

C.　Since the final image is formed by diverging light rays, it is virtual.

D.　The final virtual image is erect. This is indicated by the positive sign that is given for the total magnification.

CHAPTER 6.
EQUIVALENT LENSES

1. A.　This is the same lens as in Problem 1 of Chapter 5. We have already calculated the following:

　　$P_1 = +10.40$ D

　　$P_2 = +20.80$ D

　　Equivalent power:

　　$P_e = P_1 + P_2 - cP_1P_2$

　　$P_e = 10.40$ D $+ 20.80$ D $- (0.030$ m $/ 1.52)(+10.40$ D$)(+20.80$ D$)$

　　$P_e = +26.93$ D

　　Calculation of f_e and f_e'

　　$P_e = -n / f_e = n / f_e'$

　　$+26.93$ D $= (1.00)(100) / f_e'$

　　$f_e' = +3.71$ cm

A

This distance is measured *from* the secondary principal plane, H'.

Since the lens is surrounded by air, f_e is equal to –3.71 cm. This distance is measured *from* the primary principal plane, H.

Location of principal planes:

$$\overline{A_1H} = \frac{ncP_2}{P_e}$$

$$\overline{A_1H} = \frac{(1.00)(0.030 \text{ m}/1.52)(+20.80\text{D})}{+26.93 \text{ D}} (100 \text{ cm/m})$$

$$\overline{A_1H} = +1.52 \text{ cm}$$

$$\overline{A_2H'} = \frac{-ncP_1}{P_e}$$

$$\overline{A_2H'} = \frac{-(1.00)(0.030 \text{ m}/1.52)(+10.40 \text{ D})}{+26.93 \text{ D}} (100 \text{ cm/m})$$

$$\overline{A_2H'} = -0.76 \text{ cm}$$

Calculation of P_n and P_v:

There are two approaches to calculating these values. In the first approach, we keep in mind that f_e and f_e' are measured from the principal planes, and that f_n and f_v are measured from the front and back lens surfaces, respectively.

$$f_n = -3.71 \text{ cm} - 1.52 \text{ cm}$$

$$f_n = -2.19 \text{ cm}$$

$$P_n = -n/f_n$$

$$P_n = -(1.00)(100)/-2.19 \text{ cm}$$

$$P_n = +45.66 \text{ D}$$

$f_v = 3.71$ cm $- 0.76$ cm

$f_v = +2.95$ cm

$P_v = n / f_v$

$P_v = (1.00)(100) / +2.95$ cm

$P_v = +33.90$ D

Alternatively, we can calculate F_n and F_v using the thick lens formulae:

$$P_n = \frac{P_2}{1-cP_2} + P_1$$

$$P_n = \frac{+20.80 \text{ D}}{1 - (0.030 \text{ m}/1.52)(+20.80 \text{ D})} +10.40 \text{ D}$$

$$P_n = +45.69 \text{ D}$$

$$P_v = \frac{P_1}{1-cP_1} + P_2$$

$$P_v = \frac{+10.40}{1 - (.030 \text{ m}/1.52)(+10.40 \text{ D})} +20.80 \text{ D}$$

$$P_v = +33.89 \text{ D}$$

B.   In treating the lens as an equivalent lens, distances are measured from the principal planes. The equivalent lens exists in air. As in the case of a thin lens, we ignore the lens index of refraction. If the object is located 25.00 cm from the front surface of the lens, then it is located 26.52 cm (i.e., 25.00 cm + 1.52 cm = 26.52 cm) in front of the primary principal plane. Substituting, we have:

$L' = L + P_e$

$L' = [(1.00)(100) / -25.62 \text{ cm}] +26.93$ D

$L' = +23.03$ D

$L' = n / l'$

+23.03 D = (1.00)(100) / l'

l' = +4.34 cm

This real image is located 4.34 cm to the right of the second principal plane or 3.58 cm (i.e., 4.34 cm – 0.76 cm = 3.58 cm) to the right of the second lens surface.

$M = L / L'$

M = –3.90 D / +23.03 D

M = –0.17X

(30.00 mm)(–0.17X) = –5.1 mm

This real image is inverted.

C. See the solution to Problem 1 in Chapter 5. Due to rounding, the equivalent lens approach gives a slightly different answer than the surface-by-surface approach for the image distance (measured from the back surface of the lens) and image size.

2. A. Calculate powers of two surfaces:

$P_1 = (n_L - n) / r_1$

P_1 = (1.52 – 1.00) / +0.025 m

P_1 = +20.80 D

$P_2 = (n - n_L) / r_2$

P_2 = (1.00 – 1.52) / +0.075 m

P_2 = –6.93 D

Equivalent power:

$P_e = P_1 + P_2 - cP_1P_2$

P_e = 20.80 D + (–6.93 D) – (0.010 m / 1.52)(+20.80 D)(–6.93 D)

P_e = +14.82 D

A

<u>Calculation of f_e and f_e'</u>

$$P_e = -n/f_e = n/f'_e$$

$$+14.82D = (1.00)(100) / f_e'$$

$$f_e' = +6.75 \text{ cm}$$

Since the lens is surrounded by air, f_e is equal to –6.75 cm. The secondary equivalent focal length is measured from the secondary principal plane, and the primary equivalent focal length is measure from the primary principal plane.

<u>Location of principal planes:</u>

$$\overline{A_1H} = \frac{ncP_2}{P_e}$$

$$\overline{A_1H} = \frac{(1.00)(0.010 \text{ m}/1.52)(-6.93 \text{ D})}{+14.82 \text{ D}} (100 \text{ cm/m})$$

$$\overline{A_1H} = -0.31 \text{ cm}$$

$$\overline{A_2H'} = \frac{-ncP_1}{P_e}$$

$$\overline{A_2H'} = \frac{-(1.00)(0.010 \text{ m}/1.52)(+20.80 \text{ D})}{+14.82 \text{ D}} (100 \text{ cm/m})$$

$$A_2H' = -0.92 \text{ cm}$$

<u>Calculation of P_n and P_v</u>

There are two approaches to calculating these values. In the first approach, we keep in mind that f_e and f_e' are measured from the principal planes, and that f_n and f_v are measured from the front and back lens surfaces, respectively.

$$f_n = -6.75 \text{ cm} + (-0.31 \text{ cm})$$

$$f_n = -7.06 \text{ cm}$$

$$P_n = -n/f_n$$

A

$P_n = -(1.00)(100) / -7.06 \text{ cm}$

$P_n = +14.16 \text{ D}$

$f_v = 6.75 \text{ cm} - 0.92 \text{ cm}$

$f_v = +5.83 \text{ cm}$

$P_v = n / f_v$

$P_v = (1.00)(100) /+ 5.83 \text{ cm}$

$P_v = +17.15 \text{ D}$

Alternatively, we can calculate P_n and P_v using the thick lens formulae:

$$P_n = \frac{P_2}{1-cP_2} + P_1$$

$$P_n = \frac{-6.93 \text{ D}}{1 - (0.010 \text{ m}/1.52)(-6.93 \text{ D})} + 20.80 \text{ D}$$

$$P_n = +14.17 \text{ D}$$

$$P_v = \frac{P_1}{1-cP_1} + P_2$$

$$P_v = \frac{+20.80}{1 - (.010 \text{ m}/1.52)(+20.80 \text{ D})} + (-6.93 \text{ D})$$

$$P_v = +17.17 \text{ D}$$

B.   In treating the lens as an equivalent lens, distances are measured from the principal planes. As in the case of a thin lens, we ignore the lens's index of refraction. If the object is located 15.00 cm from the front surface of the lens, then it is located 14.69 cm (i.e., 15.00 cm – 0.31 cm = 14.69 cm) in front of the primary principal plane. Substituting, we have:

$L' = L + P_e$

$L' = [(1.00)(100) / -14.69 \text{ cm}] + 14.82 \text{ D}$

$L' = -6.81 \text{ D} + 14.82 \text{ D}$

$L' = +8.01$ D

$L' = n / l'$

$+8.01$ D $= (1.00)(100) / l'$

$l' = +12.48$ cm

This real image is located 12.48 cm to the right of the secondary principal plane or 11.56 cm (i.e., 12.48 − 0.92 cm = 11.56 cm) to the right of the second lens surface.

$M = L / L'$

$M = -6.81$ D $/ +8.01$ D

$M = -0.85X$

$(10.00$ mm$)(-0.85X) = -8.50$ mm

This real image is inverted.

C.   At the first surface:

$L' = L + P$

$L' = [(100)(1.00) / -15.00$ cm$] + 20.80$ D

$L' = -6.67$ D $+ 20.80$ D

$L' = +14.13$ D

The light rays that form this image exist in glass:

$L' = n_{L} / l'$

$+14.13$ D $= (100)(1.52) / l'$

$l' = +10.75$ cm

This image is located 10.75 cm to the right of the first surface and 9.75 cm (i.e., 10.75 cm − 1.00 cm = 9.75 cm) to the right of the second surface. It serves as a virtual object for the second surface. The rays that form this virtual object exist in glass.

At the second surface:

$L' = L + P$

$L' = [(100)(1.52) / +9.75 \text{ cm}] + (-6.93 \text{ D})$

$L' = +15.59 \text{ D} + (-6.93 \text{ D})$

$L' = +8.66 \text{ D}$

The rays that form this image exist in air.

$L' = n / l'$

$+8.66 \text{ D} = (100)(1.00) / l'$

$l' = +11.55 \text{ cm}$

Magnification:

$M_T = (M_1)(M_2)$

$M_T = (-6.67 \text{ D} / +14.13 \text{ D})(+15.59 \text{ D} / +8.66 \text{ D})$

$M_T = -0.85X$

$(10.00 \text{ mm})(-0.85X) = -8.50 \text{ mm}$

Note that the surface-by-surface approach gives about the same answers as the equivalent lens approach.

CHAPTER 7.
SCHEMATIC EYES AND AMETROPIA

1. A. $100(1.00) / -6.00 \text{ D} = -16.67 \text{ cm}$

$-16.67 \text{ cm} + (-1.50 \text{ cm}) = -18.17 \text{ cm}$

$(100)(1.00) / -18.17 \text{ cm} = -5.50 \text{ D}$

To correct this myopic refractive error, the contact lens should have a power of −5.50 D.

A

B. $100(1.00) \; / \; +6.00 \; D = +16.67$ cm

16.67 cm $- \; 1.50$ cm $= +15.17$ cm

$(100)(1.00) \; / \; +15.17$ cm $= +6.59$ D

To correct this hyperopic refractive error, the contact lens should have a power of +6.59 D.

2. A. $(100)(1.00) \; / \; -7.00 \; D = -14.29$ cm

-14.29 cm $- \; (-1.50$ cm$) = -12.79$ cm

$(100)(1.00) \; / \; -12.79$ cm $= -7.82$ D

To correct this myopic refractive error, the spectacle lens should have a power of −7.82 D.

B. $(100)(1.00) \; / \; +7.00 \; D = +14.29$ cm

14.29 cm $+ \; 1.50$ cm $= +15.79$ cm

$(100)(1.00) \; / \; +12.59$ cm $= +6.33$ D

To correct this hyperopic refractive error, the spectacle lens should have a power of +6.33 D.

3. A. $A = F_{fp} + P_{eye}$

$(1.333)(1000) \; / \; a = -10.00D + 60.00 \; D$

$a = 26.67$ mm

B. $A = F_{fp} + P_{eye}$

$(1.333)(1000) \; / \; +22.22$ mm $= -10.00 \; D + P_{eye}$

$P_{eye} = +70.00$ D

4. The eye is corrected with a +5.00 D spectacle lens. What is the far point vergence that this lens produces at the cornea?

$(100)(1.00) \; / \; +5.00 \; D = +20.00$ cm

20.00 cm $- \; 1.50$ cm $= +18.50$ cm

A

$(100)(1.00) / +18.50 \text{ cm} = +5.41 \text{ D}$

$A = F_{fp} + P_{eye}$

$(1.333)(1000) / a = +5.41 \text{ D} + 60.00 \text{ D}$

$a = 20.38 \text{ mm}$

5. The patient's far point is 25.00 cm anterior to the eye, making her a –4.00 D myope as measured at the cornea. The appropriate spectacle correction is determined as follows:

$100(1.00) / -4.00 \text{ D} = -25.00 \text{ cm}$

$-25.00 \text{ cm} - (-1.50 \text{ cm}) = -23.50 \text{ cm}$

$(100)(1.00) / -23.50 \text{ cm} = -4.26 \text{ D}$

To correct this myopic refractive error, the spectacle lens should have a power of –4.26 D.

Alternatively, we can note that the far point is 23.50 cm anterior to the spectacle plane. Therefore, the spectacle correcting lens must have a power of –4.26 D to correct the ametropia.

6. The required far point vergence (at the spectacle plane) with the old correction in place is –1.00 D. Therefore, the patient's myopia will be corrected with –5.00 D spectacle lenses. The power of the contact lens required to correct the ametropia is

$(100)(1.00) / -5.00 \text{ D} = -20.00 \text{ cm}$

$-20.00 \text{ cm} + -1.50 \text{ cm} = -21.50 \text{ cm}$

$(100)(1.00) / -21.50 \text{ cm} = -4.65 \text{ D}$

7. The object produces a vergence of –6.67 D at the plane of the cornea. To compensate for this vergence, the power of the eye must either increase by +6.67 D or a lens of this power must be placed in the corneal plane. If a lens is placed in the spectacle plane, its power must be

$15.00 \text{ cm} - 1.50 \text{ cm} = +13.50 \text{ cm}$

$(100)(1.00) / +13.50 \text{ cm} = +7.41 \text{ D}$

A

To clearly see an object located 15.00 cm anterior to his cornea, this emmetrope (who can not accommodate) must look through a +6.67 D contact lens or a +7.41 D spectacle lens.

8. $L' = L + P$

$(1.333)(1000)/+24.22 \text{ mm} = [(1.000)(1000) / l] + 60.00 \text{ D}$

$l = -201.5 \text{ mm}$

The object is located 20.15 cm anterior to the cornea.

CHAPTER 8.
ACCOMMODATION

1. A. $F_{fp} = L + P_A$

     $-3.50 \text{ D} = [(1.00(100)/-10.00 \text{cm}] + P_A$

     $P_A = +6.50 \text{ D}$

The uncorrected eye must accommodate 6.50 D.

   B. $F_{fp} = L + P_A$

     $-3.50 \text{ D} = (-10.00 \text{ D} + -3.50 \text{ D}) + P_A$

     $P_A = +10.00 \text{ D}$

The eye, corrected with contact lenses, must accommodate 10.00 D.

   C.   First, find the equivalent power of the spectacle correction:

     $P = 1 / f'$

     $-3.50 \text{ D} = (1.00)(100) / f'$

     $P = -28.57 \text{ cm}$

     $-28.57 \text{ cm} - (-1.5 \text{ cm}) = -27.07 \text{ cm}$

     $P = 1 / f'$

A

$P = (1.00)(100) / -27.07$ cm

$P = -3.69$ D

Next, find the image produced by the spectacle lens:

$L' = L + P$

$L' = [(100)(1.00)/-8.50$ cm$] + (-3.69$ D$)$

$L' = -15.45$ D

$L' = 1 / l'$

-15.45 D $= (1.00)(100) / l'$

$l' = -6.47$ cm

The distance from the image to the eye is −7.97 cm [i.e., −6.47 cm + (−1.50 cm) = −7.97 cm].

Now determine the amount of accommodation required to focus the image on the retina:

$F_{fp} = L + P_A$

-3.50 D $= [(1.00)(100)/-7.97$ cm$] + P_A$

$P_A = +9.05$ D

Wearing a spectacle correction, the patient must accommodate 9.05 D.

2. First, locate the image produced by the +4.00 D contact lens:

$L' = L + P$

$L' = [(1.00)(100)/-10.00$ cm$] + 4.00$ D

$L' = -6.00$ D

$L' = 1 / l'$

-6.00 D $= (100)(1.00)/ l'$

$l' = -16.67$ cm

Next, determine the amount of accommodation required to produce the far point vergence:

$$F_{fp} = L + P_A$$

+5.00 D = [(1.00)(100)/−16.67 cm] + P_A

P_A = +11.00 D

This 5.00 D hyperopic eye, which is uncorrected by 1.00 D, must accommodate 11.00 D to focus the object onto the retina.

3. The patient can accommodate 5.00 D [(i.e., (1.00)(100)/10.00 cm − 0 = 5.00 D)]. One half of the patient's amplitude of accommodation is 2.50 D. When wearing the contact lens to view an object at a distance of 15.00 cm, the vergence leaving the contact lens must be zero.

$$F_{fp} = L + P_A$$

00.00 D = [(100/−15.00 cm) + $P_{contact\ lens}$]+ 2.50 D

$P_{contact\ lens}$ = +4.17 D

The contact lens should have a power of +4.17D. When wearing this contact lens, an object at a distance of 15.00 cm results in an image vergence of −2.50 D. The patient can see the object clearly by accommodating 2.50 D, which is one-half of his or her amplitude of accommodation.

4. $F_{fp} = L + P_A$

+2.00 D = [(1.00)(100)/−33.00 cm] + P_A

P_A = +5.00 D

Therefore, the patient's total amplitude of accommodation is 10.00 D (i.e., 2 × 5.00 D = 10.00 D).

5. Determine image location:

The object is located 11.00 cm in front of the lens (i.e., 15.00 cm − 4.00 cm = 11.00 cm).

$$L' = L + P$$

L' = [(1.00)(100)/−11.00 cm] + 1.00 D

L' = −8.09 D

A

$L' = 1 / l'$

-8.09 D $= (1.00)(100)/ l'$

$l' = -12.36$ cm

This image is located 16.36 cm [i.e., -12.36 cm $- (-4.00$ cm$) = -16.36$ cm] anterior to the cornea. The required accommodations is calculated as follows:

$F_{fp} = L + P_A$

-3.00 D $= [(1.00)(100)/-16.36$ cm$] + P_A$

$P_A = +3.11$ D

The eye must accommodate 3.11 D.

6. A. <u>Determine the image location</u>:

$L' = L + P$

$L' = [(1.00)(100)/-38.50$ cm$] + (-6.00$ D$)$

$L' = -8.60$ D

$L' = 1 / l'$

-8.60D $= (1.00)(100)/ l'$

$l' = -11.63$ cm

This image is located 13.13 cm (i.e., 11.63 cm + 1.50 cm) anterior to the cornea. The required accommodation is calculated as follows:

$F_{fp} = L + P_A$

-5.50 D $= [(1.00)(100)/-13.13$ cm$] + P_A$

$P_A = +2.12$ D

When corrected with spectacles, the eye must accommodate 2.12 D to focus an object at 40.00 cm upon the retina.

B. In LASIK, the correction occurs in the plane of the cornea. First, we determine the power of the correction that is required in the plane of the cornea:

$$P = 1 / f'$$

$$-6.00 \text{ D} = (1.00)(100) / f'$$

$$f' = -16.67 \text{ cm}$$

To correct this refractive error in the plane of the cornea, the secondary focal length of the lens must be −18.17 cm [i.e., −16.67 cm − (−1.50 cm) = −18.17 cm]. The power of the correction is:

$$P = 1 / f'$$

$$P = (1.00)(100) / -18.17 \text{ D}$$

$$P = -5.50 \text{ D}$$

The amount of accommodation required to focus an object at 40.00 cm upon the retina is calculated as:

$$F_{\text{fp}} = L + P_{\text{A}}$$

$$-5.50 \text{ D} = (-2.50 \text{ D} + -5.50 \text{ D}) + P_{\text{A}}$$

$$P_{\text{A}} = +2.50 \text{ D}$$

When corrected with LASIK, the patient must accommodate 2.50 D to focus an object at 40.00 cm on the retina.

C.   Subsequent to LASIK, the former spectacle-wearing myopic patient must now accommodate 18% more in order to see a near object. [(2.50 D − 2.12 D) (100) / 2.12 D= 18%]. This must be taken into account when counseling the patient prior to surgery and when determining the amount of correction. It may be decided to slightly undercorrect one of the myope's eyes so that this eye can be used for viewing near objects. This is referred to as *monovision*. Many but not all patients adopt to a monovision correction.

CHAPTER 9.

CYLINDRICAL LENSES AND THE CORRECTION OF ASTIGMATISM

1. A.   The vertical meridian has a power of −1.00 D and the horizontal meridian has a power of −2.00 D.

B.   −1.00 = −1.00 × 090

2. A.   The vertical meridian of the lens has a power of +6.00 D and the horizontal meridian has a power of +4.00 D. The image focused by the stronger vertical meridian will be closest to the lens.

B.   Vertically diverging light rays emitted from the object are focused closest to the lens by the stronger vertical meridian. A horizontal line that has fuzzy left and right edges is formed in this plane because the object's horizontally diverging rays are not yet focused. The upper and lower edges of this horizontal line are in focus, however, because the vertical meridian is in focus.

C. $L' = L + P$

$L' = [(1.00)(100)/−50.00 \text{ cm}] + 6.00 \text{ D}$

$L' = +4.00 \text{ D}$

$L' = 1 / l'$

$+4.00 \text{ D} = (1.00)(100)/ l'$

$l' = +25.00 \text{ cm}$

D.   At the plane where the weaker +4.00 D horizontal meridian is in focus, the rays that are focused by the vertical meridian (at 25.00 cm) are now diverging to form a vertical line. The focused horizontal rays give this vertical line sharp right and left edges. The upper and lower edges of the vertical line are fuzzy, however, because the vertical meridian is out of focus. The location of this vertical line is given by:

$L' = L + P$

$L' = [(1.00)(100)/−0.50 \text{ cm}] + 4.00 \text{ D}$

$L' = +2.00 \text{ D}$

$L' = (1.00)(100)/ / l'$

$l' = + 50.00 \text{ cm}$

E.   50.00 cm − 25.00 cm = 25.00 cm

F.   The circle of least confusion is *dioptrically* centered between the image plane of the vertical meridian and the image plane of the horizontal meridian. Its location is calculated as follows:

[(4.00 D − 2.00 D)/2] + 2.00 D = 3.00 D

This corresponds to a linear distance of 33.33 cm; the circle of least confusion is located 33.33 cm from the lens.

3. A.   The vertical meridian of the lens has a power of +5.00 D and the horizontal meridian has a power of +7.00 D. The image focused by the stronger horizontal meridian will be closest to the lens.

B.   A vertical line is formed closest to the lens. At the plane where the object's horizontally diverging light rays are focused by the stronger horizontal meridian, the vertical rays have not yet focused. These out-of-focus rays form a vertical line with fuzzy upper and lower edges. The right and left edges of this line are in focus, however, because the horizontal meridian is in focus.

C. $L' = L + P$

$L' = [(1.00)(100)/-25.00 \text{ cm}] + 7.00 \text{ D}$

$L' = +3.00 \text{ D}$

$L' = 1 / l'$

$+3.00 \text{ D} = (1.00)(100)/ l'$

$l' = +33.33 \text{ cm}$

D.   A horizontal line is formed further from the lens. At the plane where the object's vertically diverging light rays are focused by the weaker vertical meridian, the horizontal rays are out of focus—they are focused closer to the lens, at +33.33 cm. These out-of-focus rays form a horizontal line with fuzzy left and right edges. The upper and lower edges of this line are in focus, however, because the horizontal meridian is in focus.

$L' = L + P$

$L' = [(1.00)(100)/-25.00 \text{ cm}] + 5.00 \text{ D}$

$L' = +1.00 \text{ D}$

$L' = 1 / l'$

+1.00 D = (1.00)(100)/ / l'

l' = +100.00 cm

E.   100.00 cm − 33.33 cm = 66.66 cm

F.   The interval of Sturm is *dioptrically* centered between the image plane of the horizontal meridian and the image plane of the vertical meridian. Its location is calculated as follows:

[(3.00 D − 1.00 D)/2] + 1.00 D = +2.00 D

This corresponds to a linear distance of +50.00 cm; the circle of least confusion is located 50.00 cm to the right of the lens.

4. A.   The vertical meridian of the lens has a power of +6.00 D and the horizontal meridian has a power of +5.00 D. Vertically diverging object rays are focused by the stronger vertical meridian to form a horizontal line. The line is located at

$L' = L + P$

L' = [(1.00)(100)/−40.00 cm] + 6.00 D

L' = +3.50 D

$L' = 1 / l'$

+3.50 D = (1.00)(100)/ / l'

l' = +28.57 cm

B.   Horizontally diverging object rays are focused by the weaker horizontal lens meridian to form a vertical line. The line is located at

$L' = L + P$

L' = [(1.00)(100)/−40.00 cm] + 5.00 D

L' = +2.50 D

$L' = 1 / l'$

+2.50 D = (1.00)(100)/ / l'

l' = +40.00 cm

C.   40.00 cm − 28.57 cm = 11.43 cm

D.   [(3.50 D − 2.50 D)/2] + 2.50 D = 3.00 D

Therefore the circle of least confusion is located 33.33 *cm* from the lens.

5. A.   The vertical meridian of the lens has a power of +4.00 D and the horizontal meridian has a power of +6.00 D. Horizontally diverging object rays are focused by the stronger horizontal meridian to form a vertical line. The line is located at

$$L' = L + P$$

$$L' = [(1.00)(100)/-40.00 \text{ cm}] + 6.00 \text{ D}$$

$$L' = +3.50 \text{ D}$$

$$L' = 1 / l'$$

$$+3.50\text{D} = (1.00)(100)/ / l'$$

$$l' = +28.57 \text{ cm}$$

B.   Vertically diverging rays are focused by the weaker vertical lens meridian to form a horizontal line. The line is located at

$$L' = L + P$$

$$L' = [(1.00)(100)/-40.00 \text{ cm}] + 4.00 \text{ D}$$

$$L' = +1.50 \text{ D}$$

$$L' = 1 / l'$$

$$+1.50 \text{ D} = (1.00)(100)/ / l'$$

$$l' = +66.67 \text{ cm}$$

C.   66.67 cm − 28.57 cm = 38.10 cm

D.   [(3.50 D − 1.50 D)/2] + 1.50 D = 2.50 D

Therefore the circle of least confusion is located 40.00 cm to the right of the lens.

6. A.   +10.00 = −14.00 × 090; −4.00 = +14.00 × 180

B.   +10.00 = −10.00 × 090; pl = +10.00 × 180

C.   +5.00 = −8.00 × 180; −3.00 = +8.00 × 090

D.   +2.00 = −8.00 × 090; −6.00 = −8.00 × 180

7. A.   Against-the-rule compound hyperopic.

B.   With-the-rule compound myopic astigmatism.

C.   With-the-rule mixed astigmatism.

8. Both meridians of the eye are focused anterior to the retina. The vertical bars are focused by the horizontal meridian. Since these bars are clearer than the horizontal bars, they (the vertical bars) are focused closest to the retina. The more blurred horizontal bars are focused by the stronger vertical meridian anterior to the focus of the vertical bars. The astigmatism is therefore with-the-rule.

CHAPTER 10.
PRISMS

1. A. $n \sin \theta_1 = n' \sin \theta'_1$

$(1.00)(\sin 30.0°) = (1.52)(\sin \theta'_1)$

$\theta_1' = 19.2°$

The deviation produced by the first surface (β_1) is:

$30.0° - 19.2° = 10.8°$

B. $\alpha = \theta'_1 + \theta_2$

$60.0° = 19.2° + \theta_2$

$\theta_2 = 40.8°$

$n \sin \theta_2 = n' \sin \theta'_2$

$(1.52) \sin 40.8° = (1.00) \sin \theta'_2$

$\theta_2' = 83.3°$

The deviation produced by the second surface (β_2) is:

$83.3° - 40.8° = 42.5°$

C. $\beta = \beta_1 + \beta_2$

$\beta = 10.8° + 42.5°$

$\beta = 53.3°$

or,

$\beta = \theta_1 + \theta_2{}' - \alpha$

$\beta = 30.0° + 83.3° - 60.0°$

$\beta = 53.3°$

2. $P_P = (100)(\tan \sigma)$

$P_P = (100)(4.0 \text{ cm}/500 \text{ cm})$

$P_P = 0.8\ ^\Delta$

3. $P_P = (100)(\tan \sigma)$

$15.00\ ^\Delta = (100)(2.00 \text{ cm}/d)$

$d = 13.3 \text{ cm}$

4. $P_P = (d_{cm})(P)$

$P_P = (0.50 \text{ cm})(8.00 \text{ D})$

$P_P = 4.0\ ^\Delta$

Remember, when using Prentice's rule, d is in centimeters.

5. $P_P = (d_{cm})(P)$

$2.0\ ^\Delta = (d_{cm})(6.00 \text{ D})$

$d = 0.33 \text{ cm or } 3.3 \text{ mm}$

Remember, when using Prentice's rule, d is in centimeters.

A

6. $(1.00)(100) / -13.00$ cm $= -7.69$ D. The prism does not change the vergence of the light rays that are incident upon it.

7. A. $n \sin \theta_1 = n' \sin \theta'_1$

       $(1.00)(\sin 45.0°) = (1.52)(\sin \theta'_1)$

       $\theta'_1 = 27.7°$

       $\alpha = \theta'_1 + \theta_2$

       $84.0° = 27.7° + \theta_2$

       $\theta_2 = 56.3°$

       $n \sin \theta_2 = n' \sin \theta'_2$

       $(1.52) \sin 56.3° = (1.00) \sin \theta_2'$

       $\theta'_2 > 90.0°$

    B.   Total internal reflection occurs at the second surface (see Chap. 1).

CHAPTER 11.

DEPTH OF FIELD

---

1. Since the hyperfocal distance is 200.00 cm, the total depth of field is 1.00 D. If the near point of accommodation is 10.00 cm, the true amplitude of accommodation is 9.50 D (i.e., 10.00 D − 0.50 D = 9.50 D).

2. First, we calculate the true amplitude of accommodation. The patient's range of clear vision (at near) corresponds to a dioptric range of 1.00 D to 4.00 D. Since the depth of field is 1.00 D, the true amplitude of accommodation is 2.00 D (i.e., 3.00 D − 1.00 D = 2.00 D). When looking through the distance prescription, the patient can accommodate 2.00 D. If the depth of field was zero, the patient could not resolve objects nearer than 50.00 cm. The near boundry of the patient's range of clear vision, however, is extended by one-half of the depth of field (i.e., 0.50 D). Therefore, the range of clear vision through the distance portion of the spectacles is from infinity to 40.00 cm (i.e., −2.50 D). [Due to depth of field, when the patient is focused at 50.00 cm (−2.00 D) she can see clearly at 40.00 cm (−2.50 D).]

A

3. The far point for an uncorrected 1.00 D myope is –1.00 D. Due to depth of field, which is centered at a distance of 100.00 cm, the patient can see clearly out to a distance of –0.25 D or 400.00 cm (i.e., 1.00 D – 0.75 D = 0.25 D).

4. Through the add, the patient can see clearly out to 50.00 cm. Since the depth of field is 0.50 D, the patient's add has a power of +2.25 D (i.e., 2.00 D + 0.25 D = 2.25 D). In other words, when a +2.25 D lens focuses the eye at 44.44 cm, the patient's depth of field allows her to see out to 50.00 cm.

Another approach to solving this problem is to first determine the true amplitude of accommodation. The dioptric range of clear vision is from 2.00 to 5.00 D. Since 0.50 D of this range is due to depth of field, the patient's amplitude of accommodation is 2.50 D. If there were no depth of field, the patient would need an add of 2.50 D to see at 20.00 cm (5.00 D –2.50 D = 2.50 D). Taking into account depth of field, however, we know the power of the patient's add is only 2.25.

5. The true amplitude of accommodation is

(5.00 D – 2.50 D) – 0.75 D = 1.75 D

Without spectacles, the 4.00 D myope's eyes are focused at 25.00 cm. Combined with accommodation and depth of field, the uncorrected patient has a near point of:

4.00 D + 1.75 D + 0.75/2 D = 6.13 D.

This corresponds to a linear distance of 16.33 cm.

6. The uncorrected eye is focused at 3.00 D. For the range of clear vision to extend from 4.00 to 2.00 D, the depth of field must be a total of 2.00 D. In looking through the 2.00 D add, the furthest distance at which objects can be resolved is

2.00 D – 1.00 D = 1.00 D or 100.00 cm.

In looking through the add fully accommodated, the near boundary of the patient's range of clear vision is

2.00 D + 2.00 D + 1.00 D = 5.00 D, or 20.00 cm

The linear range of clear vision through the add is 100.00 to 20.00 cm.

A ───────────

1. A. $M_{ang} = -P_2 / P_1$

$M_{ang} = -(+25.00 \text{ D}) / (+10.00 \text{ D})$

$M_{ang} = -2.5X$

If the Keplerian telescope contains an erecting element, the magnification is +2.5X.

B. The focal length of the objective lens is 10.00 cm and the focal length of the eyepiece (ocular) is 4.00 cm. Therefore, the tube length is 14.00 cm (i.e., 10.00 cm + 4.00 cm = 14.00 cm).

2. The angular magnification of the telescope (ignoring signs) is

$M_{ang} = P_2 / P_1$

or

$M_{ang} = (1/f_2) / (1/f_1)$

$M_{ang} = f_1 / f_2$

$5 = f_1 / f_2$

or

$5f_2 = f_1$

From Figure 12-5A, we see that the separation of the lenses in a Galilean telescope is equal to $f_1 - f_2$. For this telescope,

$0.100 \text{ m} = f_1 - f_2$

Substituting, we have

$0.100 \text{ m} = 5f_2 - f_2$

$f_2 = 0.025 \text{ m}$

and

$5f_2 = f_1$

$5(0.025 \text{ m}) = f_1$

$f_1 = 0.125 \text{ m}$

Therefore

$P_1 = +8.00 \text{ D}$

$P_2 = -40.00 \text{ D}$

(We know that the second lens is negative because the system is Galilean.)

3. A. Image formation by the objective:

$L' = L + P$

$(1.00)(100)/l' = [(1.00)(100)/-100.00 \text{ cm}] + 8.00 \text{ D}$

$l' = +14.29 \text{ cm}$

Since the lenses are separated by 10.00 cm, this image is 4.29 cm to the right of the eyepiece. It serves as a virtual object for this lens.

$L' = L + P$

$L' = [(1.00)(100)/+4.29 \text{ cm}] + (-40.00 \text{ D})$

$L' = -16.69 \text{ D}$

B. If the light entering the telescope has zero vergence, then the light leaving it will also have zero vergence. In viewing an object at a distance of 100.00 cm, a +1.00 D lens cap results in light rays of zero vergence entering the telescope.

4. A. The patient can read the material if it is 3X closer to the eye ($6M/2M = 3X$), at a distance of 13.3 cm (40.0 cm / 3 = 13.3 cm). This is the equivalent viewing distance. The patient could hold the material 13.3 cm from her eye or at the focal point of a lens that has an equivalent viewing power of about +7.50 D (100 / 13.3 cm ~ 7.50 D).

B. Since the reading material is held at the focal point of the magnifying lens, the retinal image size is the same regardless of the distance between

A

the magnifying lens and the eye. The patient can hold the lens at the distance from the eye that she finds most comfortable.

C.   Increased magnification can be obtained if the patient looks through the magnifying lens with her add, *and* the distance between the add and the magnifier is less than the focal length of the magnifying lens.

5. For the patient to read 1 M print, the print must be held 5X closer than the original reading distance of 40.0 cm. The equivalent viewing distance is therefore 8.0 cm (40.0 cm / 5 = 8.0 cm), and the equivalent viewing power is +12.5 D. If the patient holds reading material at the focal point of a +12.50 D lens, the rays emerging from the plus lens are parallel and focused onto the retina when the patient views through the distance portion of his spectacles.

6. A.   The equivalent viewing distance is 13.3 cm. Since the telescope has an angular magnification of 2.0X, the reading material can be held twice as far away—at 26.6 cm—and still subtend the same angle. For the light rays that enter the telescope to be parallel, the reading material must be held at the focal point of a lens cap with a power of ~ +3.75 D (i.e., 100 / 26.6 cm ~ +3.75 D).

Let us solve this problem using a slightly different approach. For the patient to read 2 M print, the print must be enlarged by a factor of 3.0X. Since the telescope provides magnification of 2.0X, the lens cap must provide the remaining magnification of 1.5X (3.0 / 2.0 = 1.5X). To do so, the reading material must be held 1.5X closer than the original distance—it must be held at 26.7 cm (40.0 cm / 1.5 = 26.7 cm). When an object is at the focal point of a +3.75 D lens cap (100 / 26.7 cm ~ 3.75 D), parallel light rays enter the telescope.

B.   The reading material should be at the focal point of the lens cap.

C.   The telemicroscope has a narrow field of view, permitting the patient to see only a limited portion of the reading material.

CHAPTER 13.
RETINAL IMAGE SIZE

1. Prior to LASIK, there was only 2.00 D of (refractive) anisometropia; consequently it made little difference if the correction was in the form of spectacles or contact lenses. (Theoretically, contact lenses would result in the two eyes having equal image sizes, since the ametropia is refractive.) Following

A

the procedure, there is 5.00 D of refractive anisometropia, making the form of the correction more important. Based only on considerations of retinal image size, a contact lens should be prescribed for the left eye.

2. Retinal image size in corrected ametropia:

$$y'' = \frac{-\theta}{P_L + P_{eye} - dP_L P_{eye}}$$

Since the ametropia is corrected with contact lenses, d is zero and the power of the correcting lens (P_L) is equal to the far point vergence (F_{fp}). Substituting, the above equation can be rewritten as

$$y'' = \frac{-\theta}{F_{fp} + P_{eye}}$$

Applying the principles of lens effectivity, we know that the ametropia can be corrected with the following contact lens prescription:

OD −5.50 DS

OS −2.87 DS

Substituting in the above equation, the retinal image size in the right eye (corrected with a contact lens) is

$$y'' = -\theta / (-5.50 \text{ D} + 60.00 \text{ D}) = -\theta / 54.50 \text{ D}$$

and the retinal image size in the left eye (corrected with contact lens) is

$$y'' = -\theta / (-2.87 \text{ D} + 60.00 \text{ D}) = -\theta / 57.13 \text{ D}$$

Using the right eye as the comparison standard, the percentage difference in the uncorrected retinal image sizes is

Percentage difference =

$$\frac{(-\theta/57.13D) - (-\theta/54.50D)}{-\theta/54.50D} (100)$$

A

Percentage difference = −4.6%. The retinal image of the left eye is 4.6% smaller than the retinal image of the right eye.

3. $\theta'/\theta = 1 / (1-dP_L)$

For a +7.00 DS lens:

$\theta'/\theta = 1 / [(1 - (0.015\ m)\ (+7.00\ D] = 1.12X$

For a +1.00 DS lens:

$\theta'/\theta = 1 / [(1 - (0.015\ m)\ (+1.00\ D] = 1.02X$

The percentage difference is

$[(1.02 - 1.12) / 1.12]100 = -8.93\%$

The angular magnification produced by the left lens is 8.93% less than that produced by the right lens.

CHAPTER 14.
REFLECTION

1. A. $P = -2 / r$

$P = -2 / -0.30\ m$

$P = +6.67\ D$

$L' = L + P$

$L' = [(1.00)(100)/-5.00\ cm] + 6.67\ D$

$L' = -13.33\ D$

$L' = -1 / l'$

$-13.33\ D = -(1.00)(100) / l'$

$l' = +7.51\ cm$

Since the image vergence is negative, the image is formed by diverging light rays and is virtual.

A

$M = L / L'$

$M = -20.00 \text{ D} / -13.33 \text{ D}$

$M = +1.50X$

$(2.00 \text{ cm})(+1.50) = +3.00 \text{ cm}$

The image is erect.

2. A. $P = -1 / f'$

$P = -1 / +0.15 \text{ m}$

$P = -6.67 \text{ D}$

$L' = L + P$

$L' = [(1.00)(100)/-25.00 \text{ cm}] + (-6.67 \text{ D})$

$L' = -10.67 \text{ D}$

$L' = -1 / l'$

$-10.67D = -(1.00)(100) / l'$

$l' = +9.37 \text{ cm}$

B.   Since the image vergence is negative, the image is formed by diverging light rays and is virtual.

$M = L / L'$

$M = -4.00 \text{ D} / -10.67 \text{ D}$

$M = +0.37X$

$(2.00 \text{cm})(+0.37X) = +0.74 \text{ cm}$

The image is erect.

3. Since the image is real and 40.00 cm from the mirror, the image vergence is +2.50 D.

$L' = L + P$

+2.50 D = L + 30.00 D

L = −27.50 D

$L = 1 / l$

−27.50 D = (1.00)(100) / l

l = −3.64 cm

Since the object vergence is negative, the object is real. It is located 3.64 cm to the left of the mirror.

4. Since the image is virtual and 10.00 cm from the mirror, the image vergence is −10.00 D.

$L' = L + P$

−10.00 D = L + −30.00 D

L = +20.00 D

$L = 1 / l$

+20.00 D = (1.00)(100) / l

l = +5.00 cm

Since the object vergence is positive, the object is virtual (i.e., a virtual object). It is located 5.00 cm to the right of the mirror.

5. A.   We will solve this problem with two different approaches. First, we treat the optical system surface-by-surface. The light rays that emerge from the source are first refracted by the lens, then reflected by the mirror, and once again refracted by the lens.

Refraction at lens:

$L' = L + P$

L' = [(1.00)(100)/−20.00 cm] + 15.00 D

L' = +10.00 D

$L' = 1 / l'$

$+10.00 \text{ D} = (1.00)(100) / l'$

$l' = +10.00 \text{ cm}$

This image is located 7.00 cm to the right of the mirror (i.e., 10.00 cm − 3.00 cm = 7.00 cm). It serves as a virtual object for the mirror:

$L' = L + P$

$L' = L + (-2/r)$

$L' = (1.00 /+0.07 \text{ m}) + (-2/+0.02 \text{ m})$

$L' = 14.29 \text{ D} + (-100.00 \text{ D})$

$L' = -85.71 \text{ D}$

$L' = -1 / l'$

$-85.71 \text{ D} = -(1.00)(100) / l'$

$l' = +1.17 \text{ cm}$

The virtual image (formed by diverging rays) is located 1.17 cm to the right of the mirror and 4.14 cm to the right of the lens (1.17 cm + 3.00 cm = 4.17 cm). This image serves as a real object for the lens. (The light rays incident on the mirror are reflected back through the lens.) Since the reflected light rays travel from right to left, we cannot use our linear sign convention. Rather, we use absolute values.

$| L | = | 1/ l |$

$| L | = | 100 / 4.17 \text{ cm} |$

$L = -23.98 \text{ D}$

$L' = L + P$

$L' = -23.98 \text{ D} + 15.00 \text{ D}$

$L' = -8.98 \text{ D}$

This virtual image is located 11.13 cm to the right of the lens.

Alternatively, we can construct an equivalent mirror and use this mirror to determine the image distance.

First, locate the surface of equivalent mirror:

$|L| = |1/l|$

$|L| = |100 / 3.00 \text{ cm}|$

$L = -33.33 \text{ D}$

$L' = L + P$

$L' = -33.33 \text{ D} + 15.00 \text{ D}$

$L' = -18.33 \text{ D}$

The surface of the equivalent mirror is located 5.46 cm to the right of the lens.

Now, let us locate the center of curvature of the equivalent lens:

$|L| = |1/l|$

$|L| = |100 / 5.00 \text{ cm}|$

$L = -20.00 \text{ D}$

$L' = L + P$

$L' = -20.00 \text{ D} + 15.00 \text{ D}$

$L' = -5.00 \text{ D}$

The center of curvature of the equivalent lens is located 20.00 cm to the right of the lens or 14.54 cm to the right of the surface of the equivalent mirror (20.00 cm − 5.46 cm = 14.54 cm).

The power of the equivlent mirror is

$P = -2 / r$

$P = -2 / .1454 \text{ cm}$

$P = -13.76 \text{ D}$

The object is located 25.46 cm in front of the surface of the equivalent mirror (20.00 cm + 5.46 cm = 25.46 cm).

$L' = L + P$

$L' = (100 / -25.46 \text{ cm}) + (-13.76 \text{ D})$

$L' = -17.69 \text{ D}$

This virtual image is located 5.65 cm to the right of the surface of the equivalent mirror or 11.11 cm to the right of the lens (5.65 cm + 5.45 cm = 11.11 cm). This is about the same as we found with the surface-by-surface approach.

B.   Surface-by-surface approach:

$M_T = (M_1)(M_2)(M_3)$

$M_T = (-5.00 \text{ D} / +10.00 \text{ D})(+14.29 \text{ D}) / (-85.71 \text{ D})(-23.98 \text{ D}/-8.98 \text{ D})$

$M_T = +0.22X$

Equivalent-mirror approach:

$M_T = L / L'$

$M_T = -3.93 \text{ D} / -17.69 \text{ D}$

$M_T = +0.22X$

6. $P = -2 / r$

$P = -2 / +0.0078 \text{ m}$

$P = -256.41 \text{ D}$

$L' = L + P$

$L' = [(1.00)(100)/-10.00 \text{ cm}] + (-256.41 \text{ D})$

$L' = -266.41 \text{ D}$

$L' = -1 / l'$

$-266.42 \text{ D} = -(1.00)(1000) / l'$

$l' = +3.75 \text{ mm}$

Purkinje image I is located 3.75 mm to the right of the cornea.

7. Relative to the vertical meridian, the horizontal meridian of the cornea minifies the image. Therefore the horizontal meridian is stronger and the patient has against-the-rule astigmatism.

8. The keratometry readings show that the horizontal meridian is stronger than the vertical meridian, making the corneal astigmatism against-the-rule. Also, by drawing a lens cross for the patient's prescription, we see that the horizontal meridian of the eye has more power (i.e., it requires a weaker hyperopic correction) than the vertical meridian.

9. $FR = [(n' - n) / (n' + n)]^2$

   A. $FR = [(1.62 - 1.00) / (1.62 + 1.00)]^2$

       $FR = 0.056$

       Percentage reflected is 5.6%

   B. $FR = [(1.50 - 1.00) / (1.50 + 1.00)]^2$

       $FR = 0.04$

       Percentage reflected is 4.0%

   C.   The higher index lens because more light is reflected by this surface.

   D. $n_c = (n_g)^{1/2}$

       $n_c = (1.62)^{1/2}$

       $n_c = 1.27$

10. A.   The lens is fitted on flat K. The correction required in that meridian (i.e., the horizontal meridian) is −3.00 D. Therefore, the required contact lens power is −3.00 DS. The fluid lens will correct the corneal astigmatism.

   B.   The lens is fitted one diopter steeper than flat K. The correction required in that meridian (i.e., the horizontal meridian) is −3.00 D plus −1.00 D to correct for the +1.00 D fluid lens caused by the steepness of the lens. Therefore, the required contact lens power is −4.00 DS. The fluid lens will correct the corneal astigmatism.

   C.   The correction in the horizontal meridian must be −3.00 D. If the contact lens has a power of −2.50 DS, it must be fitted 0.50 D flatter than flat

K: it must have a base curve of 41.50 D. The fluid lens will correct the corneal astigmatism.

11. The amount of corneal toricity (correction), in minus cylinder form, is −2.00 DC × 090. By multipling this value by 1.25 and adding −0.50 DC × 090, Javal's rule gives the estimated amount of ocular astigmatism in the spectacle plane as −3.00 DC × 090.

12. A.   To arrive at −5.00 DC × 090 of ocular astigmatism in the spectacle plane, the corneal toricity (correction) must be −3.60 × 090. The horizontal meridian must have a K reading of 47.60.

B.   The corneal toricity is against-the-rule.

CHAPTER 15.
ABERRATIONS

1. A.   Due to spherical aberration, the subject will see two point images.

B.   When the subject occludes the top hole, the upper image disappears. The rays entering the top hole are focused on the inferior portion of the retina and are seen as the upper image. (Assumes positive spherical aberration.)

2. LASIK flattens the central cornea, thereby increasing the amount of positive spherical aberration.

3. A.   No, because the Siedel aberrations can not be corrected by a spherical lens or surface. Siedel aberrations are present with a spherical optical system.

B.   Yes, if the lens is custom-made for a particular eye and does not rotate. The lens would be nonspherical.

4. A.   If we ignore the thickness of the lens, we can assume that both the front and back surfaces of the lens have a power of +2.50 DS. The radius of curvature for the front surface is

$$P = (n' - n) / r$$

$$+2.50 \text{ DS} = (1.50 - 1.00) / r$$

$$r = +0.20 \text{ m, or } +20.00 \text{ cm}$$

A

Therefore r_1 = +20.00 cm and r_2 = −20.00 cm.

$X = (r_2 + r_1) / (r_2 − r_1)$

$X = (−20.00 \text{ cm} + 20.00 \text{ cm}) / (−20.00 \text{ cm} − 20.00 \text{ cm})$

$X = 0$

B. Plano-convex.

C. The plano surface should face the patient's eye.

5. A. $V = (n_d − 1) / (n_f − n_c)$

Glass 1:

$V = (1.59 − 1.00) / (1.61 − 1.57)$

$V = 14.75$

Glass 2:

$V = (1.73 − 1.00) / (1.76 − 1.70)$

$V = 12.17$

Also

$P_1 / V_1 = −P_2 / V_2$

$P_1 / 14.75 = −P_2 / 12.17$

$P_1 = −1.21 P_2$

And

$P_t = P_1 + P_2$

$+10.00 \text{ D} = −1.21 P_2 + P_2$

$P_2 = −47.62 \text{ D}$

But

$P_1 = −1.21 P_2$

$= (−1.21)(−47.62 \text{ D})$

P_1 = +57.62 D

B.   Calculate the radius of first surface, which has a power of +28.81 D (+57.62 D / 2 = +28.81 D):

$P = (n' - n) / r$

+28.81 D = (1.59 − 1.00) / r

r = +0.0205 m, or +2.05 cm

Since the first lens is equiconvex, the second surface of the lens has a radius of curvature of −2.05 cm. The first surface of the second lens must also have a radius of −2.05 cm. The power of this surface in air is

$P = (n' - n) / r$

P = (1.73 − 1.00) / −0.0205 cm

P = −35.61 D

Therefore the power of the back surface of the second lens is

−47.62 D = −35.61 D + P

P = −12.01 D

The radius of this surface is

$P = (n' - n) / r$

+12.01 D = (1.00 − 1.73) / r

r = +0.0608 m, or +6.08 cm

6. $\omega = (n_f - n_c) / (n_d - 1) = 1 / V$

ω = 1 / 14.75

ω = 0.068

7. $d = (f_1' + f_2') / 2$

d =[(1.00)(100)/+7.00 D + (1.00)(100) /+4.00 D] / 2

d = 19.64 cm

Index

Note: Page numbers followed by *f* indicate figures; those followed by *n* indicate footnotes; those followed by *t* indicate tables.

A

Abbe's number, 245
Accommodation, 95–110, 96*f*, 97*t*
    amplitude of, 96, 97*t*, 152
    in corrected ametropia, 103–108,
        104*f*, 106*t*, 107*f*
    definition of, 95
    in emmetropic eye, 96–98, 97*f*, 98*f*
    near point of, 101, 102*f*, 103
    presbyopia correction and, 108–110,
        109*f*, 110*f*
    in uncorrected ametropia, 98–100,
        99*f*–101*f*
Achromatic doublets, 245
Achromatic lenses, chromatic optical
    aberrations and, 245–247, 246*f*
Adaptive optics, 241
Afocal optical systems, 171
Against-the-rule astigmatism, 123
Airy's disks, 148, 149*f*
Ametropia, 87. *See also* Astigmatism;
        Hyperopia; Myopia; Presbyopia
    corrected
        accommodation in, 103–108, 104*f*,
            106*t*, 107*f*
        angular size of retinal image in,
            183–184
        physical size of retinal image in,
            184–187, 185*f*, 186*f*, 187*t*

Ametropia, corrected (*cont.*)
        laser and surgical correction of,
            schematic eyes and, 90–92,
            93*f*
    uncorrected
        accommodation in, 98–100,
            99*f*–101*f*
        linear size of retinal image in,
            179–181, 180*f*, 181*t*
Amplitude of accommodation, 152
Angle kappa, 207
Angle of deviation of prisms, 133–135,
    134*f*
Angle of refraction, 6, 8–9, 9*f*–11*f*
Angular magnification
    in corrected ametropia, 183–184
    with plus lenses, 162–163
    of telescopes, determination of,
        173–174, 174*f*, 175*t*
Anisometropia, 183
Anterior nodal point, 73, 74*f*
Antireflective coatings, 203–206, 204*f*,
    205*f*
Asthenopia, 95
Astigmatism, 113–130, 114*f*
    classification of, 123–125, 124*f*, 125*f*
    image formation and
        extended sources and, 121–123,
            122*f*

point sources and, 119, 120*f*, 121
Astigmatism (*cont.*)
  Jackson crossed-cylinder test for,
    126*f*, 126–127, 128*f*
  lens crosses and, 114*f*, 114–116,
    115*f*
  lens formulae/prescriptions for,
    116–118, 117*f*, 118*f*
  patient's vision with, 129–130, 130*f*
  radial (marginal; oblique), optical
    aberrations and, 234*f*, 234–235,
    235*f*
  spherical equivalency and, 127, 129,
    129*f*
Astronomical telescopes, 172*f*, 173
Axial hyperopia, 85
Axial myopia, 82

B
Back vertex focal length, 64, 66
Back vertex power of equivalent
    lenses, 66–67, 70, 71*f*
Barrel distortion, 236, 237*f*
Base curve, 214–215
Bending factor, 227
Best corrected acuity, 159
Bifocal adds, 96, 108–110, 109*f*, 110*f*
  determining power of, 152, 154
  magnifying lenses in combination
    with, 166–167
Blur circles, 145, 146*f*, 147*f*, 147–148,
    149*f*

C
Cardinal points, 74
Catoptrics, 196*n*
Center of curvature, 13, 14*f*
Chromatic optical aberrations, 225,
    243–248, 244*f*
  achromatic lenses and, 245–247,
    246*f*
  dispersive power and constrigence
    and, 244–245
  of human eye, 247–248, 248*f*
  lateral (transverse), 249, 250*f*
  red-green refraction technique and,

248*f*, 249–250
Circle of least confusion, 121
Classic aberrations, 226–227
  of human eye, 237–238
Closed-circuit television (CCTV), as
    magnifier, 170
Coma (optical aberration), 229–230,
    233*f*
Concave mirrors, ray tracing and, 191,
    193, 193*f*, 194*f*
Constrigence, chromatic optical
    aberrations and, 245
Contact lenses
  keratometry and, 214–216, 217*f*,
    218*f*, 219, 220*f*
  retinal image size and, 186–187
Converging pencils, 2, 3*f*
Converging surfaces, vergence
    relationship and, 32–34, 33*f*
Convex mirrors, ray tracing and, 193,
    195*f*
Corneal topography, 207, 213–214,
    214*f*–216*f*
Critical angle, 9, 10*f*
Curvature of field, optical aberrations
    and, 235, 236*f*
Cylindrical lenses, 113, 114*f*, 115
  prescriptions for, 116

D
Deformable mirrors, 239, 241, 243*f*
Depth of field, 145–156, 146*f*
  blur circles and visual acuity and,
    145, 147*f*, 147–148, 149*f*
  depth of focus and, 150*f*–153*f*,
    150–152, 154
  hyperfocal distance and, 154*f*–156*f*,
    154–155
Depth of focus, 150*f*–153*f*, 150–152,
    154
Diffraction, 148, 149*f*
Diffraction pattern, 148
Diopters (D), 4–5, 5*f*, 28
Dioptrics, 196*n*
Dispersion, 244
Dispersive power, chromatic optical
    aberrations and, 244–245

Distortion, 236, 237*f*
Diverging pencils, 2, 3*f*
Diverging surfaces, vergence
   relationship and, 35–37, 36*f*
Duochrome test, 248*f*, 249–250

E
Effective magnification, 160–162, 161*f*
Electromagnetic radiation, 1, 2*f*
Emmetropia
   accommodation and, 96–98, 97*f*, 98*f*
   schematic eyes and, 79*f*, 79–80
      far point and, 85
Entrance pupils, 173–174, 174*f*
Equivalent focal length, 63
Equivalent lenses, 63–74
   back vertex power of, 66–67, 70,
      71*f*
   definitions related to, 63*f*, 63–64, 65*f*
   equivalent power of, 64–66, 67, 69
   front vertex power of, 66, 69–70,
      71*f*
   image vergence and, 71
   locating images using, 72*f*, 72–73
   nodal points and, 73–74, 74*f*
   principal planes of, 67, 68*f*
Equivalent mirrors, 209, 210*f*, 211,
   212*f*, 213
Equivalent power of equivalent lenses,
   64–67, 69
Exact eye, 77, 78*f*
Exit pupils, 173–174, 174*f*
Exophoria, prisms for, 140, 142, 142*f*,
   143*f*
Extended objects, 2, 3*f*
Extrafocal distances, 50

F
Far point of eye, 80–81, 82*f*
Far-point vergence relationship,
   schematic eyes and, 83, 85–87,
   86*f*, 87*f*
Field
   curvature of, 236, 236*f*
   depth of. *See* Depth of field
Fixed-focus stand magnifiers, 167,

168*f*, 169–171
Fluid lenses, 216, 218*f*
Focal lengths
   back vertex, 64, 66
Focal lengths (*cont.*)
   equivalent, 63
   front vertex, 63–64, 66
   primary, 16, 18
   refracting power and, 18–19, 19*f*
   secondary, 14, 19
Focal points
   location of, vergence relationship
      and, 35
   primary, 16*f*, 16–18, 17*f*
   secondary, 13, 14*f*, 15
   for thin lenses, 43–44, 46*f*, 47, 47*f*
Focus, depth of, 150*f*–153*f*, 150–152,
   154
Frequency, 1
Front vertex focal length, 63–64, 66
Front vertex power of equivalent
   lenses, 66, 69–70, 71*f*
Fundus imaging, monochromatic
   optical aberrations and, 242, 242*f*

G
Galilean telescopes, 171, 172*f*
Gullstrand #1 model, 77, 78*f*
Gullstrand #2 model, 77, 78*f*

H
Hartmann-Shack aberrometer,
   238–239, 240*f*
Hirschberg test, 207, 208*f*
Hyperfocal distance, 154*f*–156*f*,
   154–155
Hypermetropia, 83*n*
Hyperopia, 83–85, 84*f*
   axial, 85
   corrected, accommodation in, 106*t*,
      106–108, 107*f*
   refractive, 85
   schematic eyes and, 82–85, 83*f*, 84*f*
   uncorrected, accommodation in,
      99–100, 100*f*, 101*f*

I

Image formation
  in astigmatism, 123–125, 124*f*, 125*f*
Image formation (*cont.*)
  by spherocylindrical lenses, 119,
    120*f*, 121
    extended sources and, 121–123,
      122*f*
Images
  locating using equivalent lenses, 72*f*,
    72–73
  real, 21–22, 22*f*
  retinal, size of, 179–188
    angular magnification in corrected
      ametropia and, 183–184
    linear, in uncorrected ametropia,
      179–181, 180*f*, 181*t*
    physical, in corrected ametropia,
      184–187, 185*f*, 186*f*, 187*t*
    spectacle magnification and,
      181–183, 182*f*
  virtual, 22–23, 23*f*
Image vergence, equivalent lenses and,
  71
Index of refraction, 6, 8*t*
Internal reflection, total, 9, 10*f*
Interval of Sturm, 121
Irregular astigmatism, 123

J

Jackson crossed-cylinder (JCC) test,
  126*f*, 126–127, 128*f*
Javal's rule, 219, 221, 222*f*

K

Keplerian telescopes, 171, 172*f*, 173
Keratometry, 207
  contact lenses and, 214–216, 217*f*,
    218*f*, 219, 220*f*
Knapp's law, 186
K readings, 214, 215

L

Laser-assisted in situ keratomileusis
  (LASIK), 91–92, 93*f*
Lateral chromatic optical aberrations,
    250, 251*f*
Lateral magnification, 34
  with plus lenses, 159–160, 160*f*, 161*f*
Lateral spherical aberrations, 227
Law of reflection, 191
Lens caps for telescopes, 174–176,
    175*f*, 176*f*
Lens capsule, 95
Lens crosses, 114*f*, 114–116, 115*f*
Lens effectivity, schematic eyes and,
    87–90, 88*f*, 90*f*–92*f*
Lenses
  achromatic, chromatic optical
      aberrations and, 245–247, 246*f*
  contact
    keratometry and, 214–216, 217*f*,
      218*f*, 219, 220*f*
    retinal image size and, 186–187
  cylindrical, 113, 114*f*, 115
    prescriptions for, 116
  equivalent. *See* Equivalent lenses
  fluid, 216, 218*f*
  meridians of, 113, 114*f*, 115, 115*f*
  plus, 159–163
    angular magnification with,
      162–163
    effective magnification with,
      160–162, 161*f*
    lateral magnification with,
      159–160, 160*f*, 161*f*
    prescribing, 163–166, 165*f*
    problems with, 163
  prismatic effects of, 137, 137*f*–139*f*
  size, 183
  spherical
    prescriptions for, 116
    refractive power of, 113, 114*f*
    spherical equivalent, 127, 129,
      129*f*
  spherocylindrical, 114–116, 115*f*
    extended sources and, 121–123,
      122*f*
    image formation by, 119, 120*f*,
      121
    prescriptions for, 116–118, 117*f*,
      118*f*
  thin, 43–51, 44*f*, 45*f*
    focal points for, 43–44, 46*f*, 47,

47*f*
   multiple-surface optical systems
     and, 53–57, 55*f*, 57*f*
   Newton's relation and, 50–51, 51*f*
Lenses, thin (*cont.*)
   ray tracing and, 47, 48*f*
   vergence relationship and, 47, 49*f*,
     49–50
Light
  definition of, 1, 2*f*
  point sources of, 2, 3*f*
  vergence of, 4*f*, 4–5, 5*f*
Light rays, 2, 3*f*
  convergence of, 13–15, 14*f*
  divergence of, 15, 15*f*
Linear magnification. *See* Lateral
   magnification
Longitudinal chromatic aberration, 244
Longitudinal spherical aberration, 227,
   231*f*
Low vision, 159

M
Magnification
  angular
    in corrected ametropia, 183–184
    with plus lenses, 162–163
    of telescopes, determination of,
      173–174, 174*f*, 175*t*
    spectacle, 181–183, 182*f*
Magnifiers, 159–166
  closed-circuit television as, 170
  fixed-focus stand magnifiers as, 167,
    168*f*, 169–171
  magnifying lenses and bifocal adds
    in combination as, 166–167
  plus lenses as, 159–163
    angular magnification with, 162–163
    effective magnification with,
      160–162, 161*f*
    lateral magnification with,
      159–160, 160*f*, 161*f*
    prescribing, 163–166, 165*f*
    problems with, 163
  telescopes as, 170–176
    angular magnification by,
      determining, 173–174, 174*f*,

175*t*
    Galilean, 171, 172*f*
    Keplerian, 171, 172*f*, 173
    lens caps for, 174–176, 175*f*, 176*f*
Marginal astigmatism, optical
   aberrations and, 234*f*, 234–235,
   235*f*
Meiosis, senile, 147
Meridians, 113, 114*f*, 115, 115*f*
  astigmatism classified by, 123
Minus-cylinder form of lens
   prescriptions, 117*f*, 117–118, 118*f*
Minus surfaces, 15
Mires, 214, 217*f*
Mirrors
  concave, ray tracing and, 191, 193,
    193*f*, 194*f*
  convex, ray tracing and, 193, 195*f*
  deformable, 239, 241, 243*f*
  equivalent, 209, 210*f*, 211, 212*f*, 213
  plane, ray tracing and, 195–196,
    196*f*
  power of, 196–198, 198*f*
Monochromatic optical aberrations,
   225, 238–243, 240*f*, 241*t*, 242*f*
  fundus imaging and, 242, 242*f*
  supernormal vision and, 239, 241,
    243*f*
Multiple-surface optical systems,
   53–61, 54*f*
  thick lens, 59*f*, 59–61
  thin lens, 53–57, 55*f*, 57*f*
  virtual objects and, 57–59, 58*f*
Myopia
  axial, 82
  corrected, accommodation in, 104*f*,
    104–106, 106*t*
  night, 238
  refractive, 82
  schematic eyes and, 80–82, 81*f*, 82*f*
  uncorrected, accommodation in, 99

N
Near point of accommodation (NPA),
   101, 102*f*, 103
Negative relative accommodation
   (NRA), 109

Negative surfaces, 15
Neutralizing power of equivalent
    lenses, 66, 69–70, 71*f*
Newton's relation, thin lenses and,
    50–51, 51*f*
Night myopia, 238
Nodal points, equivalent lenses and,
    73–74, 74*f*
Nonspecular surfaces, 191, 192*f*

O

Objects, 2
    extended, 2, 3*f*
Object vergence, 56, 58
Oblique astigmatism, 123
    optical aberrations and, 234*f*,
        234–235, 235*f*
Optical aberrations, 225–251
    chromatic, 225, 243–248, 244*f*
        achromatic lenses and, 245–247,
            246*f*
        dispersive power and constrigence
            and, 244–245
        of human eye, 247–248, 248*f*
        lateral (transverse), 249, 250*f*
        red-green refraction technique
            and, 248*f*, 249–250
    coma, 229–230, 233*f*
    curvature of field and, 235, 236*f*
    distortion, 236, 237*f*
    monochromatic, 225, 238–243, 240*f*,
        241*t*, 242*f*
        fundus imaging and, 242, 242*f*
        supernormal vision and,
            240, 242*f*
    paraxial assumption and, 225–226,
        226*f*
    radial (oblique; marginal) astigmatism
        and, 234*f*, 234–235, 235*f*
    Seidel (classic), 226–227
    of human eye, 237–238
    spherical, 227–229, 228*f*–233*f*
    wavefront sensing and, 237
Optical axis, 13
Optical center, 73

P

Parallel pencils, 2, 3*f*
Paraxial assumption, optical
    aberrations and, 225–226, 226*f*
Paraxial relationship. *See* Vergence
    relationship
Pencils (light rays), 2, 3*f*
Perfectly diffusing surfaces, 191
Photons, 1–2
Photorefractive keratotomy (PRK), 91,
    93*f*
Pincushion distortion, 236, 237*f*
Pinhole effect, 147
Pinholes for visual acuity testing, 145,
    147*f*, 147–148, 149*f*
Plane mirrors, ray tracing and,
    195–196, 196*f*
Plano, 114, 114*f*
Plus-cylinder form of lens prescriptions,
    116, 117*f*, 117–118, 118*f*
Plus lenses, 159–163
    angular magnification with, 162–163
    effective magnification with,
        160–162, 161*f*
    lateral magnification with, 159–160,
        160*f*, 161*f*
    prescribing, 163–166, 165*f*
    problems with, 163
Plus surfaces, 13
Point sources of light, 2, 3*f*
Polychromatic light, aberrations and.
    See Chromatic optical aberrations
Positive relative accommodation
    (PRA), 110
Positive surfaces, 13
Power
    of mirrors, 196–198, 198*f*
    of prisms, 135–136, 136*f*
Power factor in spectacle magnification,
    181–182, 182*f*
Prentice's rule, 137, 139*f*, 139–140,
    141*f*
Presbyopia, 95. *See also* Bifocal adds
    absolute, 145, 146*f*
    correction of, 108–110, 109*f*, 110*f*
Primary equivalent focal length, 63
Primary focal length, 16, 18
Primary focal points, 16*f*, 16–18, 17*f*
Principal planes of equivalent lenses,
    67, 68*f*

Prisms, 133–143, 134*f*
  angle of deviation and, 133–135, 134*f*
  clinical applications of, 140, 142, 142*f*, 143*f*
Prisms (*cont.*)
  power of, 135–136, 136*f*
  Prentice's rule and, 137, 139*f*, 139–140, 141*f*
  prismatic effects of lenses and, 137, 137*f*–139*f*
Purkinje (Purkinje-Sanson) images, 206*t*, 206–213, 207*f*, 208*f*, 217*f*
  location of Purkinje image I and, 207, 208*f*, 209
  location of Purkinje image III and, 209, 210*f*, 211, 212*f*, 213

Q
Quanta, 1–2

R
Radial astigmatism, optical aberrations and, 234*f*, 234–235, 235*f*
Radial keratotomy (RK), 91, 93*f*
Radius of curvature, 19
Ramsden circles, 173
Ray tracing, 191, 193–196
  with concave mirrors, 191, 193, 193*f*, 194*f*
  with convex mirrors, 193, 195*f*
  with plane mirrors, 195–196, 196*f*
  thin lenses and, 47, 48*f*
Real images, 21–22, 22*f*
Red-green refraction technique, 249*f*, 249–250
Reduced eye model, 77, 78*f*
Reference distance, magnification and, 160
Reflection, 191–222, 192*f*
  antireflective coatings and, 203–206, 204*f*, 205*f*
  corneal topography and, 213–214, 214*f*–216*f*
  internal, total, 9, 10*f*

Javal's rule and, 219, 221, 222*f*
  keratometry and contact lenses and, 214–216, 217*f*, 218*f*, 219, 220*f*
  law of, 191
Reflection (*cont.*)
  power of mirrors and, 196–198, 198*f*
  Purkinje images and, 206*t*, 206–213, 207*f*, 208*f*, 217*f*
    location of Purkinje image I and, 207, 208*f*, 209
    location of Purkinje image III and, 209, 210*f*, 211, 212*f*, 213
  ray tracing and, 191, 193–196
    with concave mirrors, 191, 193, 193*f*, 194*f*
    with convex mirrors, 193, 195*f*
    with plane mirrors, 195–196, 196*f*
  vergence relationship and, 198–199, 200*f*, 201–203, 202*f*
Refracting power
  calculating, 19, 20*f*, 21
  focal lengths and, 18–19, 19*f*
Refraction, 5–6, 7*f*, 8*f*, 8*t*
  index of, 6, 8*t*
  red-green technique for, 249*f*, 249–250
  at spherical surfaces, 13–23
    calculation of refracting power and, 19, 20*f*, 21
    converging and diverging surfaces and, 13–15, 14*f*, 15*f*
    focal points and, 13, 14*f*–17*f*, 15, 16–18
    real images and, 21–22, 22*f*
    refracting power and focal lengths and, 18–19, 19*f*
    virtual images and, 22–23, 23*f*
Refractive errors, 87
Refractive hyperopia, 85
Refractive myopia, 82
Refractive power, 14–15
  of spherical lenses, 113, 114*f*
Regular astigmatism, 123
Retinal images, size of, 179–188
  angular magnification in corrected ametropia and, 183–184
  linear, in uncorrected ametropia,

179–181, 180*f*, 181*t*
physical, in corrected ametropia,
184–187, 185*f*, 186*f*, 187*t*
spectacle magnification and,
181–183, 182*f*

S

Schematic eyes, 77–93
ametropia correction and, with laser
and surgical procedures, 90–92,
93*f*
emmetropia and, 79*f*, 79–80
far point and, 85
far-point vergence relationship and,
83, 85–87, 86*f*, 87*f*
Gullstrand #1 model, 77, 78*f*
Gullstrand #2 model, 77, 78*f*
hyperopia and, 82–85, 83*f*, 84*f*
lens effectivity and, 87–90, 88*f*,
90*f*–92*f*
myopia and, 80–82, 81*f*, 82*f*
reduced eye model, 77, 78*f*
Secondary equivalent focal length, 63
Secondary focal length, 14, 19
Secondary focal point, 13, 14*f*, 15
Secondary nodal point, 73, 74*f*
Seidel aberrations, 226–227
of human eye, 237–238
Senile meiosis, 147
Shape factor
meanings of, 227*n*
in spectacle magnification,
181–183
Sign conventions, vergence relationship
and, 31–32, 32*f*
Simplified eye, 77, 78*f*
Size lenses, 183
Snell's law, 6, 8–9, 9*f*–11*f*
Spectacle magnification, 181–183, 182*f*
Specular surfaces, 191, 192*f*
Spherical aberrations, 227–229,
228*f*–233*f*
Spherical equivalent lenses, 127, 129,
129*f*
Spherical lenses
prescriptions for, 116
refractive power of, 113, 114*f*
spherical equivalent, 127, 129, 129*f*

Spherical surfaces, refraction at. *See*
Refraction, at spherical surfaces
Spherocylindrical lenses, 114–116, 115*f*
image formation by, 119, 120*f*, 121
prescriptions for, 116–118, 117*f*, 118*f*
Standard distance, magnification and,
160
Stand magnifiers, fixed-focus, 167,
168*f*, 169–171
Supernormal vision, monochromatic
optical aberrations and, 240, 242*f*

T

Telemicroscopes, 175–176, 176*f*
Telescopes, 170–176
angular magnification by,
determining, 173–174, 174*f*,
175*t*
Galilean, 171, 172*f*
Keplerian, 171, 172*f*, 173
lens caps for, 174–176, 175*f*, 176*f*
Television, closed-circuit, as magnifier,
170
Terrestrial telescopes, 172*f*, 173
Thick lens formulas, 65–66
Thick lens multiple-surface optical
systems, 59*f*, 59–61
Thin lenses, 43–51, 44*f*, 45*f*
focal points for, 43–44, 46*f*, 47, 47*f*
Newton's relation and, 50–51, 51*f*
ray tracing and, 47, 48*f*
vergence relationship and, 47, 49*f*,
49–50
Thin lens multiple-surface optical
systems, 53–57, 55*f*, 57*f*
Topographic maps, 214, 216*f*
Total internal reflection, 9, 10*f*
Transverse chromatic optical
aberrations, 249, 250*f*
Transverse magnification. *See* Lateral
magnification

V

Vergence, 4*f*, 4–5, 5*f*
Vergence changer, 27
Vergence relationship, 27–40, 29*f*, 30*f*
converging surface and, 32–34, 33*f*

diverging surface and, 35–37, 36*f*
far-point, schematic eyes and, 85–87,
  86*f*, 87*f*
focal point location and, 35
locating objects with given image
  location and, 37–38, 38*f*
optical aberrations and, 225–226,
  226*f*
Vergence relationship (*cont.*)
  reflection and, 198–199, 200*f*,
    201–203, 202*f*
  sign conventions for, 31–32, 32*f*
  surface with no power and, 38–40,
    39*f*
  thin lenses and, 47, 49*f*, 49–50
Vertex distance, 88*n*

Vertex power
  back, of equivalent lenses, 66–67,
    70, 71*f*
  front, of equivalent lenses, 66–67,
    70, 71*f*
Virtual images, 22–23, 23*f*
Virtual objects, multiple-surface optical
  systems and, 57–59, 58*f*
Visual acuity
  best corrected, 159
  testing, 145, 147*f*, 147–148, 149*f*
V-value, 245

W
Wavefront sensing, 237
Wavelength, 1
With-the-rule astigmatism, 123

Z
Zernicke polynomials, 239, 241*t*